The Orange Wire Problem and
Other Tales from the Doctor's Office

the
orange wire
problem
and other
tales from
the doctor's
office

David Watts

University of Iowa Press
Iowa City

University of Iowa Press, Iowa City 52242

Copyright © 2009 by the University of Iowa Press

www.uiowapress.org

Printed in the United States of America

Design by April Leidig-Higgins

The University of Iowa Press is a member of Green Press Initiative and is committed to preserving natural resources.

Printed on acid-free paper

Library of Congress Cataloging-in-Publication Data
Watts, H. David.
The orange wire problem and other tales from the doctor's office / by David Watts.
     p.   cm.
Includes bibliographical references.
ISBN-13: 978-1-58729-800-4 (pbk.)
ISBN-10: 1-58729-800-7 (pbk.)
1. Physician and patient — Anecdotes.   2. Medicine — Anecdotes.   3. Physicians — Anecdotes.   I. Title.
R727.3.W383 2009   2008035418
610.69'6 — dc22

09 10 11 12 13 C 5 4 3 2 1

For Joan

*The really good witch
doctor puts a drop
of his own blood in
the potion.*

Contents

Acknowledgments

"Thank You Mr. Nicholson" appeared in the *San Francisco Chronicle Magazine*, June 5, 2005.

The poems in "A Critical Distance" were first published in *Blessing* (Barnwood Press, 2003).

Mary Oliver's poem "Wild Geese" is from *Dream Work*, copyright © 1986 by Mary Oliver. Used by permission of Grove/Atlantic, Inc.

"The Pill on the Shelf," "Brilliance," and "Thank You Mr. Nicholson" have been aired as commentary on National Public Radio's *All Things Considered*.

Preface | What You Might Expect to Find Here

Truth be known, doctors are, shall we say, strange people. Oh, to be sure, they may be wonderful, even magnificent at times, but the way they think can make us wonder, occasionally, if they just got off the spaceship from Pluto.

It has something to do with training, I think — all that science and very little humanity. It has to do with daily doses of death and disease, needing to ride above it all while harboring a schizophrenic split between engagement and safe distance. It comes from living constantly in a community of high expectation and a limit to the knowledge we have. Innovation, free thinking, and even quirky behaviors become necessary orders of the day if we are to land on a pathway to healing.

While all this is going on, here we are, trying to act confident and trustworthy. If we weren't strange to begin with, we'd soon get that way.

In bits and pieces, largely from interacting openly with my patients and their struggles, I have come to know my insanities, some innate, some acquired, and to accept them like a father his own progeny. In this book you will see in projections upon the screen of human interactions what has resulted from this enterprise, at least as it appears from one doctor's perspective, and how the inner workings of a doctor all click together. Or don't.

Such high levels of complexity and tension produce rather unexpected outcomes at times. And praise be for that. Break points are reached where solutions arrive like blessings that are neither earned nor logical but seem somehow to work, points where what we thought was so important becomes secondary, where the characteristics of the new situation could not have been predicted from the elements that created it — one cannot always explain how we arrive or why what works, works. But you've got to pay attention.

The doctor-patient relationship is like a poem in the making. If the poet listens, the poem will tell you where it wants to go. Forced, it falls apart. Once the technique of science is brought into the healing process the beauty and shape of the outcome derives from the listening. This combination of craft and openness to the element of surprise gives us a chance to be rewarded along the way with these little unexpected epiphanies.

How best to say all this? Why, of course, by telling stories.

So that's what's in this book, stories about a doctor and his patients and the mysterious, quirky connections we make when suddenly faced with mortality and find ourselves way off the road map, alone and distressed. Emergencies like these open the lid on the curious clockwork we hide inside.

Why stories? Well, for centuries stories have, by context and example, taught us many things. In the unique circumstance of a visit to the doctor rare windows sometimes open and shine briefly upon the naked human spirit. One must choose carefully how to speak of this. Not, certainly, by cold analysis. What is needed is not so much that which dissects and reduces but that which sums up the generous and complex layers and, in the process, reveals something to us.

These stories are true — better stated, they come as close to truth as words and memory and protection of identity allow. I'm told that makes them nonfiction essays, and I suppose people do have to decide where on the shelf to put a book such as this, next to Twain or would it be Oliver Sacks . . . ? Yet to me these little sums strive not so much to document as to approach a truth that goes beyond nonfiction and dares to flirt with the realm of mystery, for indeed there is more mystery in the union between doctors and patients than a good spelunker could bring forth with a lot of time, a long rope, and a very bright light.

At a jazz concert recently I was admiring how effortlessly the musicians moved among notes and phrases to produce a rich and exciting sound. So many choices. How tight the ensemble. As a musician myself, I knew the jazzers couldn't make sense of melodies and harmonies unless they were spot on when it came to the theory of music. While they create what sounds like effortless tinkering, they think constantly about the direction a melodic line might take, chord structures, chord progressions, which inversions to play, which chords resolve naturally to other chords, whether to add a seventh or a ninth, how long to sustain *dissonance* before rewarding the ear with *harmony*. It's art, to be sure, but it's *art against the backdrop of science.*

How like the practice of medicine that is, knitting together something artistic while thinking how to push down the cholesterol, how to support the blood vessels that struggle against the damaging effects of elevated blood pressure, how to balance the loss of a vital spark of personality against the favorable effects of controlling Parkinson's a little better . . . Medicine, more than one might think, depends upon *improvisation*. This idea is hard to show by any chemical formula or didactic lecture.

I was taught that doctors imperil their decision-making process if they are on familiar terms with their patients. I have experienced exactly the opposite.

My mentor, Dr. John Carbone, was renowned for his personable manner. One afternoon he admitted one of his patients to the hospital and was making his way to the bedside when he discovered a third-year medical student well into the second hour of a long and tedious interview, a practice that in teaching hospitals trains new physicians and produces long and tedious notes in the chart.

Dr. Carbone excused himself and sat on the edge of the bed. After a lighthearted conversation he placed his hand on the arm of his patient and said, Now Mr. Roberts, I don't want you to worry about this surgery tomorrow. You're going to do just fine. With that, he stood up and walked out the door.

The patient smiled, turned to the medical student, and said, Isn't that Dr. Carbone just wonderful? He spends so much *time* with his patients.

Dr. Carbone had been there maybe three minutes; the medical student, centuries. But whatever that Carbone quality was, it had made Mr. Roberts's time with him seem expansive with layers and chambers.

Science keeps most but not all doctors from being quacks. Yet the sheer volume of material that gets forced into our brains leaves little room for balance. We list to one side when we walk. Distance swells between knowledge and wisdom, and the missing link is perspective. Stories can help that.

Stories about what works and doesn't work teach us how to stay centered. After all, we have to balance new thinking, improvisation, science, art, and a personal touch and do so in a different and challenging way with each and every patient. Stories remind us what is important about all this in a manner reminiscent of Tolstoy's three questions:

What is the most important time?
Now. No other time matters.
Who is the most important person?
The one you are with.
What is the most important thing to do?

Tolstoy answers this question: "making that person, the one standing at your side, happy." The answer he demonstrates in his story is to do good for that person.

To answer our original question, what you might expect to find here is a careful attempt to find truths we cannot find any other way, to record mystery, to discover how closely we are connected to each other, and to celebrate the sometimes quirky, offbeat behaviors that lead to pathways out of the maze. I've learned a lot writing these stories, and this above all: The doctor-patient relationship is a rare moment. It is a privilege and an honor to be part of it. I know of nowhere else we can so quickly set aside inhibitions and talk about matters of the deepest importance. Maybe that's it. Maybe what attracts storytellers is that rare opportunity to trace the mysterious movements of the human spirit and, if we're lucky, lift suffering into art, dissonance into music.

The Orange Wire Problem and
Other Tales from the Doctor's Office

Facts and Lies

Well, your pulse is great. The emergency room nurse is bending over my foot, his tattooed deltoid rippling with fine movements of support for the hand that reaches to feel my ankle. His words, the last to come from the ER staff after a six-hour visit, are, I assume, intended to reassure, which they do, arriving like carriers of some thread of connection between us, a fellowship perhaps, a gesture both well intended and well received. And I *do* feel better, better able to face the tremors in my muscles, fatigued by hours of clenching a tight protection for the red-hot joint, now diminishing after the long needle's nip, the suck-out of orange reticulated fluids and the push of Novocain and steroids to soothe the singe. I am in the aftermath, in the place where the body luffs in its wheelchair like sails in a dying wind. And here, in this place, his words *do* mean something to me, even though I know he's lying.

You see, the problem is he palpated the wrong place, not behind the *inside* of my ankle, where the posterior tibial artery runs like a river of renewal, but — a common mistake — behind the *outside*, where it does not. That he chose to tell me the pulse was great even though he didn't feel it — couldn't possibly have felt it — let me know he meant to say something grander, maybe something that sounds more like best wishes or you're going to be all right.

What puzzles me is that even though I knew his mistake as he was making it, that contrary knowledge did not prevent the good deed from happening or being well received. I'm a doctor, for Christ's sake. A scientist. I know that he was lying, and, even knowing the lie, the lie still landed its effect. What *was* it, then, given the factual error he'd made, that kept this interchange from disaster?

Here was this macho kind of guy who'd just finished dressing me again around the searing pain of my swollen joint — this pox of ingratitude I received like a Job's carbuncle for trying to rescue my son — who probably didn't need rescuing in the first place — rescue him from the ski accident I *imagined* he was about to have, and, in my awkward fatherly haste, crossed skis with him. Hours later the crystalline ooze of malevolence that comes along with the fangs and grip of that obscure condition called pseudogout starts its sinister little game — all this has landed me securely in the wheelchair, where I was to wait another hour to be picked up, trembling in the aftermath of pain and exhaustion — his report on the status of my pulse floating in like a gesture only part of a larger gesture that signaled something to me — maybe only that I was being cared for. For although skill and accuracy were missing, *intention* was there. And somehow intention was enough.

So here I sit not minding the chill of my body so much, not minding the wait so much, sustained at least partly by the effort, though flawed, the nurse had made to try and make me feel better.

And for whatever the hell reason, I do.

The Orange Wire Problem

He is the best physician who
is the best inspirer of hope.

— JOHN KEATS

It's the Orange Wire Problem, he said. Then he leaned back in his camp chair and looked me straight in the eye, raising one eyebrow in a manner intended to say that, beyond question, everyone should know what the Orange Wire Problem is.

In this way he put me at a calculated disadvantage, simultaneously in a state of deficiency and curiosity. I now possessed the best combination of qualities for an audience about to be abused by a storyteller.

Dinner and dominoes had been cleared away, and the fire was crackling in the pit beyond our tired, rapacious feet. Though a member in good standing in this men's club for many years, I am seldom present at these late-night gatherings, partly because I am busy being busy, partly because I felt it strange to socialize without women present. What keeps me coming back is the opportunity to play the great classics in the club orchestra, where I play French horn, and the slow discovery that men in the absence of women are very different animals. They can actually be quite interesting. Without the drive for female attention men relax and open up a bit.

It's one of the fundamental ideas of the universe, he said, half figuring we thought he was lying, half tantalizing us with a possible truth.

Then, as bait, he left a little agitated silence that called forth a feeling of awkwardness, knowing what was expected, knowing he required some kind of gesture to entreat him — just a little playful begging before he'd consent to go on.

I bit the bait. What is? I said.

Let me tell you about this, he said.

By this time of the encampment we'd already had the long dinner-table talks we always have about chemistry and health. Nicolas is a brilliant engineer, quick, authoritative, and, at the same time, an outspoken medical agnostic. Something in his past made him distrust doctors and the stuff they spew they call science. He took as his hero not James Watson or Francis Crick but Andrew Weil. He surfs the Net. He comes up with all the cancer preventatives and cures that sound, on the surface, astounding but, as I occasionally point out, lack the science to hold water.

Whereupon we would discuss again the opposing truths of Koch's postulates — the cornerstones of science, which hold that anything true is only observable as true in a strictly controlled circumstance and that it must, in identical circumstances, be able to be reproduced exactly — scientific method, in a word, as opposed to the art of empirical observation. I myself am a poet and somewhat of a doubter, one who has recognized the inadequacy of science as it is currently imagined to explain all the mysteries of the universe, and so Nicolas knew he had in me an audience that would not reject him outright.

Milk thistle. Nicolas was taking inordinate amounts of milk thistle based upon some uncontrolled observations that it was supposed to be good for the liver. It has always struck me as curious that, to use Andrew "Pop" Ivy and Linus Pauling as examples, brilliance in one area of science guarantees no safe passage to another. Pop with his Krebiozen, Linus with his vitamin C, and now Nicolas, a hard science engineer with his milk thistle. To be sure, there are, hidden within the urges and intuitions of alternative medicine, clues to the truths we seek, but, paradoxically, there is in the minds of great thinkers a nodule of inclination like a blind spot, which, when emotionally engaged, will switch on an inexplicable suspension of critical thinking.

Nicolas settled in. His audience settled in.

It promised to be an adventure into the intuitive.

My friend built a car, he said. From the nuts up. I watched him out in his backyard with parts spread all around, smoking like meteors from a lava shower. Months this way he was out there tinkering and swearing.

Nobody moved. Nick was on a roll.

It was an obsession. He skipped meals, missed meetings, let the phone ring . . . Finally, in springtime, he finished. A glimmering red Maserati-like *bitch* of a car — and he'd built every goddamn inch of it.

I went out with him. Towed it to a spot in the country with a lot of road and not a lot of cops. Fired it up, and it ran great! Topped out at a hundred ten. Only one problem . . .

Now if I'd been able to move my eyes at this point, I would have seen that our circle had grown, attracting other listeners like tufts of lint to a ball of static electricity.

Everything was great . . . except for one little thing. Ran fine. Handled good. But as soon as the engine warmed up — he paused here for dramatic effect — it quit.

A little shock wave pushed me back in my chair. The old coot. We'd talked earlier in the day about my wife's Volkswagen Rabbit. Did the same thing. Damn inconvenient to be in the fast lane of some superhighway somewhere and have all your power go out like a snuffed candle. Dangerous, pretty damn. We'd taken it to several mechanics, and no one could find the answer. We quickly learned not to reveal this history of failure — which now like a strange and inexplicable pox seemed to spread by itself — couldn't reveal it because to do so would scare the next bunch of mechanics away. Mechanics hate to look bad, we found out. And the odds are, if other respectable mechanics haven't found the trouble, they won't find it either. The car might have been fixed by now, but by now it was a dead duck. Even the *Car Talk* guys wouldn't call us back.

Just sell it, my cycling buddy said. But the car had belonged to Joan's ex-father-in-law, and she was attached. She liked the car. Eventually, she donated it to the Kidney Foundation, since that's what the father-in-law died of. I guess it eased the pain, both ways.

Nick had heard me tell this story. He waited till now, the fox, to play out his response.

We took it to the mechanic, he said. They checked the gas cap air vent, the distributor head, spark plugs. (This was sounding very familiar.) Changed all the distributor wires. They threw up their hands.

So my friend took the car apart right down to the frame and built it back again . . . Same damn thing.

So I told him, listen, what you need is a psychic.

My friend looked at me like he was going to punch me out on the spot — and then we didn't speak to each other for a really long time. Every now and then I'd call him up and ask, *Car running?*

He'd just hang up the phone.

Eventually, he got so beat up by the failure of it all, he called me up and asked for her name.

I went with him. She said it was the orange wire.

Orange wire? Orange wire? He was furious. I built that goddamn car, he said, and there isn't a goddamn orange wire anywhere near it.

It's the Orange Wire Problem, she said.

He pushed the car into the backyard and let it sit there. He let the rain fall on it. Dogs pissed on it. *He* pissed on it.

Then the next spring, without any warning, he was out there taking it down to the nuts again. And there, my good friends, running along the chassis near the gear box was a little orange wire on its way to the fuel pump. Turns out, when the box heated up, the wire stopped conducting. You guessed the rest. He moved it over an inch, rebuilt the car, and ever since it's run like a cheetah.

Nick leaned back in his chair with an expression of "now I've done gone and got you under my thumb" on his face.

The story needed no explanation, and Nick was smart enough not to give one. He just looked up like he *knew* he got us good this time.

And that, gentlemen, he said, just to drive it home one more time, is the Orange Wire Problem.

Next morning at breakfast we returned, without a backward glance, to the usual, Nicolas saying he'd discovered that the PSA most doctors order is not the critical PSA, and how can anyone know if there is cancer there if you're dealing with inaccurate numbers in the first place?

I sort of knew what he was talking about but also sort of didn't. It's like knowing something lightly until the pressure comes hard and head-on, and then it seems nothing whatsoever is stored in those brain cells. And believe you me, it's kind of hard to fake it if it's Nicolas staring you down with his just-off-the-Internet knowledge about the pure direction of the universe.

I mumbled something that probably revealed more than I intended.

I'll bet not one doctor in ten knows what I'm talking about, he said.

On that I could agree. And did so. Intelligibly this time.

Richard looked at my plate. Speaking of doctors, he said, let's see if the doctor follows his own advice.

I was grateful for the unexpected assault.

Since when, I said, do doctors do that?

Eggs, do we see eggs? Richard jeered.

Yeah, but notice I didn't eat the yolks.

Nothing wrong with a little cholesterol. It was Nicolas, rising to my defense. You need some of that stuff for hormones and bile salts, he said. Besides, a lot of this fear of fats is just fabricated bullshit. And with that he held up a soggy piece of sausage, dipped it in his egg yolk, and chomped it down.

I was of two minds about that. He was right and not right. But it took a lot of energy to sort out what allowed some people to eat fats with relative impunity and required others to avoid them. I said something that approximated that idea and then skillfully turned the conversation to the Mozart Fifth Symphony, which we were rehearsing at the time and through which we could view together Mozart's youthful brilliance.

A month later on a routine blood test Nicolas turned out to have an elevated PSA. Three times normal, for Christ's sake. So I called him up.

Sounds like something ought to be done about a PSA like that, he said.

Yes, absolutely.

Then, because I knew he would agree in friendship and disagree in practice and run screaming from traditional medicine, I said that he should at least hear what the experts had to say.

Which experts?

I knew what he meant, but I ignored him. Well, there's a urologist here who not only is the reigning leader of prostate cancer surgery in the region but also embraces alternative methods of treatment.

No biopsy, Nick said.

No?

No.

How do you know for sure how to distinguish prostate hypertrophy from cancer?

The superspecific PSA.

I wasn't so sure how dependable that was, but on his turf he was calling the shots. Anyway, the urologist would have something to say about that.

Can I make you an appointment with this guy anyway?

Can't hurt.

No, it can't, I said. Especially since you're not going to let him go near you.

And he didn't. Oh, he went. But the advice to get biopsies and consider either radiation or surgery along with diet, meditation, and group meetings made him curdle and clabber and run the hell away.

From time to time at rehearsal I would ask if he was paying attention to the P problem.

He'd found this doctor in Boston who didn't do any of the *above* . . . and then it got real vague about what he did do. I wasn't certain if the confusion I felt arose from my unfamiliarity with the circumstance or his.

Well, as long as you're paying attention, I said.

Oh yes, I'm flying out tomorrow. Or maybe next week, depending.

Summer returned. And with it the little wildness of men running among trees.

We've got to get this domino problem solved, Nicolas said.

Nick is gifted. He could look at a line of dominoes and give you an accurate sum of the spots in the time it took to snap your fingers. He counted "tiles." He knew what was played and what was not and pretty well figured out by watching the way you played which of those remaining were in the bone pile and which were in your hand. I can beat anybody but a fool, he said.

Why not?

A fool doesn't know what he's doing. Therefore, he can't be figured out.

Men in woods. Dominoes everywhere. He'd sneak up behind me, look over my shoulder, and say, You've only got one play . . . and that wasn't it. Then he'd laugh hard and long. It *was* funny. He was either so right or so confident it didn't much matter.

The domino problem was that our camp had not won the club tournament since old Dick Foster had won it three years running back in the eighties. We've got a tradition to uphold, Nick said. There's no reason why I can't train a bunch of you luggards to be at least half-decent.

Well, everyone but that John Chambers. And he's just plain hopeless.

John was my partner at the time, sitting across the table, and that was, of course, the reason why Nick let fly.

Oh, sorry, John, he intoned, his face beaming with unrestrained glee. I didn't see you sitting there.

Yeah right, Nicolas. Right.

We hadn't talked PSA for some time now. I guess we'd shifted into that quality of interaction that falls under the heading of the unstated agreement. Which, to my mind, went something like this: I got to say what I thought, and then he went and did what he thought. That little philosophy of behavior pretty well matched the truth of the matter, and the only consolation it gave me was that it made both of us feel like we were discharging our responsibilities.

In reality, the issue found itself among the forgotten. The problem that wants to be left alone moves from center stage to a nagging afterthought. I didn't think prostate cancer when I looked at Nicolas. I wasn't in a clinical mode when discussing cholesterol at breakfast or what breadth of knowledge or lack thereof the average physician on any given Thursday is likely to possess. I didn't know what he was doing about "the problem." In short, it was history.

Summer came to its slow end. I hadn't seen Nicolas until he showed up.

Showed up unexpectedly at my office one day, saying he just didn't feel right. And thanks for seeing me so soon. And I seem to have lost a little weight. Maybe 15 pounds, not that I didn't need to lose weight, but not this way. I'm not very hungry. Pain? No, no pain. And no discomfort either. Diarrhea? No. Nausea? Well, not that I recognize. No. No bleeding. Yeah, I do pee a lot more, but only over a run of a day or two and then it's back to normal again. Well, maybe I do get up at night, but that too changes from day to day. What paleness? Oh, my hands? Well, I guess I hadn't noticed that, but up against yours I do look pretty white. Sallow you call it? I guess not having enough blood could be a reason for all this awful sluggishness I feel. Man, I'm beat.

I'm not just thinking anemia, I said, but also diabetes. That could explain the weight loss and frequent peeing.

Nicolas was taking off his shirt.

God, Nick. You've lost muscle. Look. There's nothing much here.

I stroked the bony prominence of his shoulder where the humerus bone rose through the folded planes of his deltoid muscle, now all but absent, leaving a sheaf of empty membranes like tissue paper lying wet over stone.

Diabetes can do this. And other endocrine diseases, like Cushing's, where you have too much steroid floating around. I was also thinking about catabolic states like cancer where the energy balance is so negative that even muscle gets thrown in the grinder. I didn't want to mention this just yet. The anxiety of dire possibility is horrific, while the anxiety of reality has, at least, a point of focus.

I sure as heck want to find out what's happening in your chemistries, I said. There's going to be an important clue in there somewhere. Can we get started?

I sent him to the lab for all the above and slippered in a PSA and a CEA, protein markers for cancers of the prostate and the internal organs.

Next day I called him.

Oh, you've got results already?

Yeah. Just hit my desk. We've got some strangeness here.

Some?

Diabetes for one. That blood sugar was 326.

Holy Christ!

Yeah. Real diabetes for sure. That explains a lot.

What else?

Well, I don't like the way the liver is looking. I mean, there's an elevation of alkaline phosphatase. That's risky business, and I want to arrange a CT scan, pronto. I've checked with the university hospital, but they're jammed till sometime around the 12th of Never, so I was wondering if you'd go to a local hospital nearby. Timing is important, and I don't want you or me to sit on this.

What are you thinking?

I knew that question was coming. The best kindness I could do was reveal thoughts and confusions as they came to me, show process rather than speculation.

Well, alkaline phosphatase is elevated in things that physically push the liver around . . . gallstones, fat, some rare storage diseases . . .

I left him a little time to digest all that, and then . . .

. . . but also in some cancers. I'd like to know, and I'm sure you would too, what we're dealing with, ASAP.

The CEA was off the charts — 60 where the normal was less than 5. I mentioned this but moved ahead. It was an awful lot to contemplate all at once, and I felt we had to prioritize. To move fast and keep the information breaking into the space just ahead of us. We were running, suddenly, a hell of a race.

Diabetes is the first priority. Let's get that under control and see how much that benefits us. I'll call you back.

I tried calling my diabetes expert. He works at UC. You can never reach anyone there, at least not in the first five calls. I walked over to his office and pulled him out of a teaching conference.

I'm going out of town this afternoon, he said.

Good. Then you'll have just enough time to see Nick before you go.

He looked at me with the fatigued eyes of someone who knows he's caught but doesn't want to be. Okay, he said. Four o'clock.

Then there was this matter of the astronomical CEA.

Colon, said my oncology friend. That's colon cancer until proven otherwise.

And I began thinking: when was Nick's last colonoscopy? Shit! Have we done a colonoscopy? Ah, yes, we talked about it, but he postponed because of the prostate thing. Then I realized that colon cancer didn't seem likely to me. No gastrointestinal symptoms, no pain, no bleeding. It had to be something else.

Or pancreatic, said the oncologist. Could be pancreatic. The CA 19-9 will help us on that. I asked if he could see Nicolas. Delighted. How about next Monday. That was a week away. Too long. I called up my other friend who had left the university long ago to "take care of patients for a change." I'll see him tomorrow, he said.

A curious sense of relief came over me. This was not a situation for relief. Where was that coming from? From the rapid dispatch of action? The satisfaction of a full-bore response? The quick disposition to the experts? I realized it might be because it was the nature of pancreatic cancer to come out of the blue, as unannounced as Pearl Harbor. Landing in the neighborhood of that diagnosis with all its unpredictability might be the source of this little glimmer of relief in the midst of my friend's devastation. Since pancreatic cancer cannot be detected or prevented, the possibility I had screwed up somehow had been removed. Horror has not the same acrid flavor without guilt. And I could see how easy it would be to let that sneaky little elation count for something, so I suppressed the thought. Selfish thought. We had work to do.

After seeing the diabetes guy Nick stopped by my office.

Insulin, he said.

Thank you, I said. I thought so.

I got on the phone to a nice technician at Sequoia Hospital who said she could do the CT scan the following morning if Nicolas would check in with them today. Nick left straightaway and at eight A.M. the next day was on the table. At noon when I returned from an endoscopy the faxed report greeted me at the appointment window. Where's Nick? I said.

Right behind you.

Oh, Nick.

Other patients were waiting for me to start my afternoon office. I took a quick look around and then beckoned for Nick to follow. My patients have always realized that if I interrupt someone else to deal with their urgent needs, they should damn well tolerate it when I do the same for others.

I had glanced at the first item on the list of impressions in the instant before I called Nick's name, and it had confirmed my fearful expectations. I was now faced with Nicolas *and* Elizabeth, his wife, in my exam room with just this sheet of paper that separated us from knowledge and, unread, still held captive all in the world that mattered.

We'll read it together, I said. I'm only now seeing it for the first time.

I understand, he said.

And I read: *The lung bases are unremarkable . . .*

The radiologists can look at that at the upper end of their swath, I said.

. . . There are multiple hepatic lesions consistent with malignancy, probably metastatic disease. The largest solitary lesion is in the anterior segment of the right lower lobe measuring 5 cm. There are lesions in all hepatic lobes. The gallbladder is present. There is no biliary dilatation. There is thrombus . . .

That's a clot . . .

. . . in the superior mesenteric and splenic veins.

These are big veins that come from the gut to the liver.

There is no mass in the pancreatic head or neck. The pancreatic tail is less well visualized and difficult to distinguish from the partially thrombosed splenic vein. A mass in the tail of the pancreas cannot be excluded. The spleen size is normal. There is a 2 cm low-attenuation mass in the gastrohepatic ligament superiorly consistent with an enlarged lymph node. There is no other abdominal abnormality. Survey of the bones is unremarkable.

Wow, he said.

Yeah.

Not great news.

I'm shocked, I said. And I was, if not by the diagnosis then by the magnitude, the outrageous largeness of that fucking tumor — imagine carrying all that cancer around for God knows how long and only showing telltale signs just now.

We could tell you were shocked the way you read it, he said. I guess I'm shocked too.

Nick turned and looked at Elizabeth. His eyes were tender but not frightened. Water he fought hard not to show collected at the periphery.

I'm sorry you have to go through this, he said.

Oh, Nick, it'll be all right, she said and put her arms around him.

I felt the urge to hold them both, to be a third person in the arc of their embrace, but something stronger held me in place. This was *their* time, the closing of the small cracks between them. To enter that sanctity would be to assume myself too large, too important. I stayed in my chair.

When they released each other I said, Anytime night or day give me a call.

I do have one regret, he said. I probably shouldn't have taken so much of that milk thistle.

I don't think that had anything to do with it, Nick. This is out of left field in the most left-fieldness of ways. Anyway, don't go there. You'll drive yourself crazy. Have you been exposed to any toxins?

Now there's an idea, he said. Lead. Lots of lead in the last few months, soldering all those electronic circuits.

I'll order lead levels.

We've got some thinking to do, he said.

As they started to leave I began *my* thinking. Where was this tumor coming from? What was the diabetes all about? Was the cancer hiding in that segment of pancreas that we could not see well on the CT scan? Did it replace the whole pancreas and therefore cause the diabetes? Did he have hemochromatosis? Which among all these questions really mattered now?

Oncologist #1 called. Largest goddamn CA 19-9 I've ever seen, he said — 56,636 with a normal of less than 31. In my book that would make it pancreatic.

Oncologist #2 sent me a fax. Don't forget that this could all be prostate, he said.

And I wondered how all this felt to Nick. I remembered when I had my head CT scan. When they pushed the iodine dye into my body it was a searing warmth spreading like a fiery emotion through my deepest inside. I remembered thinking that there was a separation between me and the event happening to me, even though there was no doubt it and I were in the same place at the same time. That distinction between the imagined event, in which I was at unity with the dye and its effects, and the event itself in real time gave the effect that I was an observer inside my own body. Did Nicolas feel that way?

We were lingering in the outer office. He mentioned again, no biopsy. I knew that. And I knew there would be no chemotherapy.

Maybe it's like that Orange Wire Problem, I said.

Yes, exactly, he said, and four years from now when we're all sitting around the campfire we'll remember the Orange Wire Problem...

And I thought to myself, my brother did that. Spoke of the time ahead as he was dying of lung cancer. Six months from now, he had said, we'll be glad we did all those drug therapies — as if to speak of the future laid claim to the future.

... and I want to tell you, Nick said, I've been checking up on...

... Poly-MVA.

Nick was back to see my colleague, oncologist #1, talking about Poly-MVA, and he seemed to be in relatively good spirits. We had an unbelievable weekend, he said. And I could imagine so, what with all the friends and family that had accreted around this collapsing but powerful nucleus. And then the plans about what to do.

Is that the Reno thing?

Yeah. But somebody is doing it in Santa Rosa too.

I don't know anything about it.

Palladium — essentially totally bound with alpha-lipoic acid. Extremely reactive electrically — electrons in the outer shell — disturbs reproduction of cancer cells but not normal cells. Also seems to reverse heart arteriosclerosis too.

This was sounding *too* great, but I said nothing to discourage him. I had put myself in the "trying to believe" mode. He was going to need my believing and my blessing as well as all the other forces he could muster.

Seventy percent improvement rate in metastatic cancer. It's been around since the early nineties. I heard about it at the Cancer Control Society meetings I just attended.

Sometimes the irony is too great to dare take note.

They don't like to use the word *cure*, he continued. Everybody knows that *cure* is a naughty word. So they say *remission* or something like that, but they are winking as they say it.

I knew a woman who took it, he said. The cancer started to dissolve. She stopped and it came back. Started again and got the same effect.

I didn't ask the obvious. Too many ripples on the water already. Sounds good, I said.

They are quick to admit they don't know the chemistry.

How about side effects?

He brightened. No side effects. None whatsoever.

Can't hurt, I offered.

Can't hurt. Sometimes it's not the why. What's that saying, Elizabeth? Oh yeah. *Knowing why is the booby prize.*

It would be wonderful to know why, he continued, but I'm the pragmatist in the house right now.

Elizabeth piped up. I was a little concerned about that scientific mind of his wanting to wait too long.

Yeah, Nick said, if I tell this to some of my science buddies they will give me a hard time.

He laughed . . . some of that woo-woo stuff. Speaking of that, I had an amazing experience — I'm lying down on my back and then this *incredible* warmth — and this is not my imagination — this sense of energy entering in my hands.

It was a healing circle, Elizabeth explained. I organized it Friday night. Some people who didn't even know him, all together, all across the country . . . all at the same time . . .

And I've had some healing dreams. All the metastatic nodules disappearing . . .

Well, dream work, I said.

Yeah?

It's the mind doing its work on the problems of the day. Isn't that what they say?

In some sort of perverse way, he said, this is an exciting journey. He looked around. Anyway, what's the choice? Elizabeth and I know a guy who did this stuff and got cured after a recurrence. The doctors were so upset they went back to the scans and tried to prove it wasn't there in the first place.

We all laughed.

Reminds me of the Symington story, I said.

Do I know that?

It's the guy who was absolutely convinced that Krebiozen would cure his lymphoma that his doctors had given up on. The doctors finally consented to get some — you know, the stuff that turned out to be soda bicarbonate or something — made the arrangements to fly some in. The plane got delayed, and the doctors decided to just inject water and *say* it was Krebiozen. Well, you know what happened. The tumor, a large mass in his chest, started going away.

Yeah, that's *Karl* Symington. I do know that story.

Karl Symington, the guy who did all that visualization stuff.

In that same moment I became aware that Elizabeth was a therapist and used visualization technique. Flickering at the edge of memory was Nick saying to me once that the audiotape she made for their friend with his two cancers was credited with saving his life. I was on firm ground here.

I believe that, Nick said.

Well, the doctors didn't, so they took X-ray after X-ray. Same deal. Melted away despite no "medication" being given.

Nick laughed.

Placebo, I said.

Placebo, he said. Pretty heady stuff.

Nick started talking about other things, his research project mapping the retina.

He's the genius behind all the technology, Elizabeth put in.

Then Nick turned the conversation back to alternative therapies. I remembered, he said, how someone said that our cells are the smallest units of our imagination. I was nodding my head — in a convincing manner, I hoped — and all the while thinking about the other part of the Symington story I had not wanted to tell, the part when the doctors revealed to the patient that it was just water they gave him, and following that the tumor sprung back on him like a hornet, and he died the following week.

Keep that belief system going, I advised. And I meant it. I didn't want to make the same mistake the doctors in Symington's story had made. And you'll like oncologist #1. He's got an alternative mind.

Yeah, we'll explore.

'Course, you'd bring it up anyway.

You're right, he said, laughing. He's got no choice.

And the laughter that followed was free-flowing and unself-conscious, nor was it weighted by diagnosis or fear. It flowed as if it were water rising from some deep place where it had been waiting a long time.

———

The visit lasted two hours. They looked awful coming out — bent over, eyelids drooping, you could tell the frame of their bodies crumbled under the weight of the hard truth they had to face.

I put my arm around Elizabeth. Too much? I said.

Just a candid observation, she said ...

Nick was sitting in one of the waiting room chairs, eyes closed, washed out.

... sometimes it's best not to know all the details.

Yeah, I said. Enough for a while.

You can say that again.

Go see a movie.

Which one?

Well, how about *What the Bleep?*

You know, you're the second person who has told me that.

We just saw it last night. It's all about quantum mechanics and how we don't really know what is going on in this world. How there are many possibilities that exist all at once, even in what seems to be an organized, orderly world. Then there's the interconnectedness of it all, where will and intention can have very mysterious but measurable effect. With the perspective you'd bring, it might be interesting.

Friday afternoon.

Elizabeth wants to speak to you before you leave today, my receptionist told me.

We couldn't get the PET scan, she said.

It was Friday. Weekend on rollers already.

Oh?

After we went there they told us he had to have his blood sugar a lot lower for it to work.

Oh.

Something about how it wouldn't image since the agent they use is a sugar or something.

I don't really know about that, I said.

If they had told us in advance we might have been able to do something about it. Nick got really heated up, and he kind of unloaded on them.

I don't blame him. They're not very good sometimes about telling you what is required.

We don't want to go back unless we are sure it can get done.

Absolutely. And I'm learning something here, I said. Let me call them and I'll call you back.

Twenty minutes later I called her.

The marker they use is a sugar. It won't go where they want it to unless your blood sugar is below 180. And you can't have any insulin within two hours or it will all go to the muscles.

Okay.

Sorry about the trouble.

Now we know.

How are things otherwise?

He was getting really jaundiced. His eyes were half-full with yellow. He had a chiropractic visit yesterday, and now the jaundice is all gone. Completely gone.

That's great, I said, trying not to sound like I was trying too hard.

Nick came to the phone.

Yeah, okay. Except I've had this headache the last two days.

Shit, I thought. The goddamn tumor is already in his head. Then I told myself not to jump to conclusions.

Try a little Advil, I said. Call me if you need something stronger.

Sorry to bother you on a Sunday afternoon with your kids and all.

It's all right.

I wanted to get a chair, something for Nicolas — he's so weak when he takes a bath or shower — something for him to sit down on while he's bathing. Do I need a prescription for that?

My God, I thought. He's fading fast ... if he can't manage a bath already ...

No, you can just get one from a medical supply house. Then in order to deduct it from your taxes as a medical expense I'll write you a prescription after the fact to cover it.

Will that work?

Should.

Okay, thanks. Sorry to bother.

No problem. How are you two holding up, anyway?

He's really weak. Sleep helps. But not enough.

I'll bet.

We got some good sleep the last two days. And I applied one of those Watson patches. It really helped. Once again he was really yellow before it went on and much less so after.

That's good, I said.

And it was the strangest thing. You could see the outline of the tumor around the patch.

How so?

You could see a little halo where the tumor was.

I knew I wasn't going to get a better explanation than that, so I let it be. If there was more to learn, I would learn it later.

We're going to do one of those treatments. You know, with Palladium?

Yeah.

If we start in Reno it gets under way Wednesday. If we do it in Santa Rosa it's next week.

Whatever you do, Elizabeth, don't wait too long, okay?

Got it. And sorry to bother.

Something had been nagging at me all through this encounter with Nicolas and his disease, something that, now that the hubbub had died down a bit and we were coasting till the next decision and because of the smallness of its voice, could only now be heard. How is it, this voice asks, that this man who is intelligent, health conscious, innovative . . . how can it be that he can get so full of cancer so fast?

I know some things about the biology of cancer and how some dividing times — doubling times, they call them — are faster than others — that's a given. Yet this one was beyond the pale at the very beginning. What is the relationship between this tumor and the body, Nick's body? How could the body *not know* it was there?

It made me think about the soul, or the spirit, or whatever it is that's inside us. Was this illness of the cell which is also an illness of the body also an illness of the soul? To me, Nick's soul was huge and powerful. It made a presence in the world that was recognizable and strong. Yet at least the body, the carriage of the soul, was flawed, deeply flawed, in fact, approaching failure.

Evil is the disease that does not announce itself. Evil is the kernel of disease that begins in a shadow and shows itself only when damage is beyond undoing. Illness of that design can serve itself no purpose, for it kills its host, its feeder, its habitat.

My question was, Does the host know this illness . . . and, if it knows, does it have the power to renounce it?

The lights went off on our street again — something about proclivity and the inability of the power company to intercede with the little power gremlin's clear intent to do mischief. Second time in two weeks — no power.

Time slows without the electronics we depend upon to keep us hyped in a state of frenzy. Dishes cleared as well as they can be in semidarkness, the voice of Gabriel, my just-turned-four-year-old son, asking his mother, Why is there no gravity in space? Why is invisible? Why . . . ? settling down the stairs from another part of the house, the diamond-shaped spaces between the wicker strokes in the chair back across from me never more evident than in this angular light-of-a-single-source, a candle . . . and still my question had no answer.

Five P.M. I had to take Duston to his cello lesson. Elizabeth called while we were driving there. We had been listening to the Red Sox–Yankees game, game seven of the play-off series tied at three all, at least listening to that part of the game I could negotiate between teenage songs on Radio Disney.

Nick's too jaundiced for therapy, she said. They won't take him. They say it would kill him. He needs a — what is it? — a drainage procedure.

I'll get right back to you, I said.

I called my colleague. He said he'd stent Nick right away. I called his secretary, and his secretary scheduled it for the following week. Not soon enough. Something got lost between doctor and doctor or between doctor and secretary.

Elizabeth was on the phone again and said we should be doing this as soon as possible. I said, I think — and then I paused to seriously consider her complaint — I think that's what we're doing.

Yes, you're right.

Then I remembered something.

I know a doctor who's a maniac and will probably do him right now. The maniac called me back in three minutes. I can do him today, he said. I work till ten P.M. Is he NPO?

Yes, I said, though I didn't know for sure. And, by the way, you're crazy.

Probably.

But thanks. Works for us.

The lights were still off at home. Rain was falling heavier and harder. The kind of energy that drifts through the house is not one akin to surface static but what arises out of silence and low light.

What did the soul know? And when did it know it?

I take notes. I write down questions.

Writing while it is happening means that at the end of the story, if the events turn out to be pedestrian or not so extraordinary, then some meaning must be found that makes this effort worthwhile. In that, the experience of writing is like life itself. Most events are not extraordinary, yet we are asked to find extraordinary meaning in them.

Ten P.M. and the maniac calls again.

No dilated ducts in his liver. No possibility of stenting.

Could you get interventional radiology to put one through his abdominal wall?

No ducts. Nothing to hit. I got ultrasound involved and we imaged him. The problem is that he has a huge, I mean *huge*, mass in the tail of the pancreas. All the blood vessels are either clotted off or filled with direct invasion of the cancer. And the liver — he paused to catch his breath — the liver is totally replaced by tumor.

He's jaundiced not because he's *obstructed* with tumor. He's jaundiced because *he has no liver.*

There was silence.

Sorry, he said. Nothing I could do.

Worse than I thought, I said.

What should I tell them?

They don't know?

I wanted to talk to you first.

He's an engineer. They'll want to know.

Yeah. He was impressed with all the technology and asked a lot of questions . . . was blown away by the images. He's doing some project to map the retina?

Yeah.

Impressive guy.

They've almost no time left. They've got a right to know.

My God, I was thinking, he was already a dead man when he came to see me. How he's surviving on so few liver cells I don't know. Worst of all, he's going to die before he has a chance to try his first treatment.

It was a quick workup, but it was a quicker cancer.

The Symington Fake pushed into my mind: If Nick's doctors refused to treat him, why not offer something to him in the form of a placebo? I imagined driving down to his house to see him, carrying with me a syringe filled with — what? Vitamin B_{12} maybe? Yeah, that would give it that red, medicinal color. Maybe a little something else in it for good measure — prepared to give, after discussing it with Elizabeth, a dramatic shot in the rump. Could we, in this way, unleash that mysterious force that responds only to the call of belief?

Would it be worth the price of lying to a dying man?

I realized I was faced with one of those possibilities that, if you don't take it, you'll never know if it was real or not. If you do and nothing happens, then at least it has cost nothing in the process, nothing, that is, but the indignity of deception at the deathbed. Which is worse, then, shutting out possibility with decorum or risking decorum for possibility? At what point does the likelihood of success dip so low, become so frivolous, as to make it altogether indecent?

There would surely be a price to pay for lying: perfidy. A breach of trust.

The power came on. The Red Sox brought in Embree to wrench the last Yankee from the cosmos — and damned if he didn't do it. It was a great comeback, miraculous, they were saying. Down three games to none to win four in a row, the last two at Yankee Stadium...

Is it not the healer's task, I was thinking, to keep the door open?

Especially when no one else will, especially when it is being so forcibly shut from all sides? Does the patient's trust extend only to the truth or to some absolute beyond truth that might help him out of his distress? Whatever that is, can belief call its name?

The rain had stopped by the time I drove my son to school the next morning. The air was cold — it was that shocking kind of morning that runs through your whole being, cutting against the warmth you cling to from your early-morning bath, held like a prayer inside — a morning that rings with vigor and promise. My son and I are talking about the Lapathon, the fund-raiser in which kids lap the school block as many times as they can to earn dollars for worthwhile causes.

And I'm thinking about the minor adjustment needed in my HDL cholesterol.

And Nick is dying.

His wife will be calling his daughters to say, If you want to see him, . . . his ideas of redemption lying on the shelf like unused coffee cups — the one you bought in Nashville with the picture of Johnny Cash on it, the crystal clear one from NPR, the one with the innovative bell-bottom design to keep it stable on a desk busy with soldering and invention, the one from Bali . . .

And I wondered where the power lay. There had to be one — one equal and opposite, one to neutralize this ravenous cancer.

And the morning spoke to me and it said, Go for it. It's Nick who's sick, not you. It is the purpose of the living to go on living. And I took a deep breath of cold, clear air and with it a new notion:

The problem of the orange wire was not about the orange wire, not even about the psychic who intuited it. It was about deciding how to allocate belief.

Duston wants drop-don't-stop today, which means that I will navigate my car inside the cones to be met by a greeter who will open the car door and let him out, in this case, Kathy, a den mother who loves Duston and calls him "The Answer Man" because he has one for every occasion.

Hello, Answer Man, she says.

Hello, Kathy.

Hurry along now — you don't want to be late.

I steer my car around the circle at the corner, the one between the school and the library, that convenient neighborhood street device that allows you to change direction without going out of your way to do it.

Tomorrow I will call Elizabeth. I will be ready to prepare the syringe: B_{12}, a bit of sterile water to sting a little, a medium-sized needle. I will want him to feel this one. I will drive down, listening, perhaps, to Bach preludes on my radio, the syringe sitting respectfully in its bucket of ice in the passenger's seat. I will tell him I've been thinking about the orange wire lately. He will nod or maybe say that he has too. He might say he wished it were as simple as all that. He might even say there is no orange wire, but I don't think he will. I will ask him if he wants me to give a message to the guys at the club. And he will say something like, *Count tiles, you bastards.* And then I might say we should name a domino tournament after him. Something just right, not too filled with rules and regulations. Something that allows brilliance to stretch out and get counted. And then we might sit for a while and listen for whatever sounds come our way, or we'll talk about whatever flows from being inert like this, not moving or even wanting to move in the room. And in the car, sitting in its ice, the syringe will wait, patient, respectful, filled with nothing but possibility.

Brain Damage

I can't believe you're still here, she said.

Idiocy, I said. It runs in the family.

She was referring to the fact that I was examining her throat and ears and chest for a prolonged upper respiratory infection while wearing a crutch and an arm sling. Her question, implied but not spoken, was, Why the hell don't you go home and take care of yourself?

This part's okay, I said. It's endoscopy that kills me.

You're not still doing endoscopy. Jeez, I can't believe it.

That's probably what the patients think.

I'll bet.

It's the shoulder separation, I said. Something about that torquing motion that really smarts.

She rolled her eyes. So taking it easy means doing only one endoscopy at a time.

Owww! I slumped in my chair and covered my heart. You got me!

She laughed.

Well, I said, my orthopedist told me I could stop doing endoscopies, heal quickly, and have a lot of endoscopies I'd have to do later on, or . . .

She jumped in . . . or you could do them all and heal a lot slower.

Right.

Right. So you're all crazy.

Probably.

Her eyes probed, her head waved side to side in a not entirely flattering expression of amazement.

My father is a doctor, she said. He ran the Sonoma Marathon a few years back. Ended up in the hospital at the end of the race.

I looked up from my writing. Liver failure probably — something as simple and entertaining as that.

Don't know. Just half-dead.

She paused and looked at me. Then, she said, he ran it again the next year . . .

Now it was my turn to finish the sentence . . . and ended up in the hospital at the end of the race.

Exactly!

You see — brain damage, I said. A man after my own heart.

But it doesn't stop there.

Oh no.

He's close to a congregation of praying Christians. He asked them to pray that he'd make the right decision about running the race again.

I laughed. He doesn't need prayer . . .

. . . he needs a brain, she said.

I was listening to her chest. I folded up my scope and declared with muted authority, Chest is clear. Looks like a sinus infection.

You remember, she says, I was the one who got her gut screwed up by antibiotics once before.

Yup.

What do you suggest?

Too long you've been working on this infection, I said. Headaches signal that it's getting pretty advanced. Cipro is not the first choice for this, but it's a *reasonable* choice, and it might actually do your gut some good in the process.

How so?

Changing around the flora a bit. Bug balance, you might say.

Let's do it, she said.

I started writing the prescription.

She was buttoning her blouse. What's plan B?

ENT.

What?

Ear, nose, and throat specialist.

No, I mean for you.

Oh, I don't know. My turn to pause and look at her. Maybe a brain transplant?

She laughed.

You know, I said, brain damage, brain damage.

She nodded.

Well, for one thing, I continued, pay the money, put the kids in ski school, and then don't go near them. These accidents all happen around trying to save them from some disaster I imagine is about to happen.

It's getting ridiculous.

Well, it is. This is the third time in four years that in December I've ended up with a significant injury: shoulder separation, torn Achilles tendon, or a major joint dislocation. Part of it is that I run around acting like a twenty year old. Part of it is that I think I can.

I'm sure in some realms you can.

Don't encourage me.

Well, poetry. But not small children on steep slopes, come on.

Yeah, and my body is telling me that even though *I* think I'm twenty, *it doesn't.*

A little slow to heal?

A little slow to heal.

Well, you don't really take care of yourself.

In ten more minutes —

Likely story —

I'm going home.

To probably do another project or something.

You know me too well and you don't even know me.

Yes, I do. I know one just like you.

I finished writing the prescription. Maybe this will change your gut flora in a good way, I said. Improve your attitude.

She scowled.

I sat back in my pivoting desk chair wheeled in by my assistant so as to make doctoring in my state of decrepitude at least not *appear* quite so outrageous. She had driven all the way up from Santa Cruz to see me, something about her complexity justified the effort. She was an English major, a writer, the kind of mind that knows bullshit when she sees it and doesn't hesitate to tell you about it. I was under her microscope and not the least uncomfortable about it.

Doctors make bad pilots, you know, I said. Especially if they're surgeons.

What made you think of that?

Well, this decision-making business that looks so dumb. For instance, it is said that a pilot has a shorter life expectancy if he is also a doctor.

That's ironic.

The way it's been explained to me is that the impulsive, confidence-based behavior that stops the patient from bleeding in the operating room is the same behavior that drives the doctor into the side of a mountain in the middle of a storm.

Can't fly a plane on operating room rules?

You have to stick to protocol. When a storm is coming you can't afford to believe, like you do in the OR, that you can just fly right through it.

Maybe you have to change your set of rules, Dr. Watts.

Right. And I was thinking that lately I was getting more accident prone. My hook shots from across the treatment room have not been landing in the wastebasket as often, the pencil I place on the shelf rolls off, the glass of water on the table tips when my sleeve catches hold of it. Pisses me off. Dangerous too. Accident-proneness together with risk-taking behavior is not the world's best combination.

Especially, she said, reading my mind, when you're getting older.

Just like a goddamn doctor, I said. Always with the bad news.

You need some rest.

And in that moment I thought that if I were to close my eyes, I could see myself lying up on my bed in the deep afternoon, a pillow under my knees, hands like dog paws across my chest, exhaling myself down to that thin line where sleep runs its path just beneath the surface . . .

You've lost weight, she said.

That's the pain.

Our eyes met. She wanted something more.

Pain takes away your appetite, I said.

You must change your life.

Thank you, Dr. Rilke. I will try.

Then I grinned a grin I couldn't have stopped if I'd wanted to.

And thanks for the consultation, I said.

Don't worry, she said, pausing at the door. I'll send you a bill.

Let Eagles Come

How does part of the world leave the world?
How can wetness leave water?

— RUMI

We never had a chance to talk about immortality, she said.

Let's do, I said.

She had raised her head where she sat crumpled between chair and examining table, eyes closed.

She had raised her head and smiled the Eastern European smile that came of its own will, forcing back the lips to a full set of teeth, as if this flashing smile were a takeover by some irresistible and benevolent force.

I'm dying, she said. I don't want it prolonged.

I just nodded to both assertions and to the others she had not stated.

What about this immortality? I said.

You know it's the universe, the indestructibility of the universe.

I sat quietly and waited for her to continue.

The universe is beyond our understanding. We know some things and then we stop knowing. But there is something more than just what we can know.

What do you *think?*

I think there is something more, but I don't have any opinion.

She paused. Only now did the original smile fade a little. I don't believe in God, she said. So here we are.

I felt her clean honesty cutting into the moment. To face death and not give into what for her would be wishful thinking . . .

There is something more in the human spirit, but, whether we find out or not . . . well, the body is perishable.

I'm dying. I don't want it prolonged . . .

I remembered her early visits — the smile came then as a shy statement of abstention. She didn't want much done, just to talk about things and share ideas. A little cramping, some gaseous distension — she wasn't sick then. No tests, she said. I have had a long and fruitful life. You should spend your time on more worthwhile projects. That same strong deflection was now present in the way she set aside all but the most sensible and essential.

It will be interesting to exchange some opinions, she says, but it's kind of late in the day.

Go on, I say.

But there is something more than the flesh, I can tell you that.

I'd like to know what makes you say so.

The many experiences I've had — some could be classified as miracles. I'm sure you've had experiences that are something similar.

Like what?

Well, I don't remember just now, but you come to a point and you know there is something there. You just can't bring it into consciousness.

Do you think you will have a consciousness on the other side?

No, not in this way — not individual consciousness. Too much to hope for.

You seem to have no fear.

No, because the universe is unlimited — no end. No beginning.

So you are on your way to participate in the universe?

Since I have left my wishes to be cremated and scattered in the sea, I'll be back into circulation quickly.

I nod. And I thought of the Native American tribe whose custom it was to lay the body out at the top of the mountain and let the eagles and the vultures come and pick it clean, entering bit by bit

Let Eagles Come

How does part of the world leave the world?
How can wetness leave water?

— RUMI

We never had a chance to talk about immortality, she said.

Let's do, I said.

She had raised her head where she sat crumpled between chair and examining table, eyes closed.

She had raised her head and smiled the Eastern European smile that came of its own will, forcing back the lips to a full set of teeth, as if this flashing smile were a takeover by some irresistible and benevolent force.

I'm dying, she said. I don't want it prolonged.

I just nodded to both assertions and to the others she had not stated.

What about this immortality? I said.

You know it's the universe, the indestructibility of the universe.

I sat quietly and waited for her to continue.

The universe is beyond our understanding. We know some things and then we stop knowing. But there is something more than just what we can know.

What do you *think*?

I think there is something more, but I don't have any opinion.

She paused. Only now did the original smile fade a little. I don't believe in God, she said. So here we are.

I felt her clean honesty cutting into the moment. To face death and not give into what for her would be wishful thinking . . .

There is something more in the human spirit, but, whether we find out or not . . . well, the body is perishable.

I'm dying. I don't want it prolonged . . .

I remembered her early visits — the smile came then as a shy statement of abstention. She didn't want much done, just to talk about things and share ideas. A little cramping, some gaseous distension — she wasn't sick then. No tests, she said. I have had a long and fruitful life. You should spend your time on more worth-while projects. That same strong deflection was now present in the way she set aside all but the most sensible and essential.

It will be interesting to exchange some opinions, she says, but it's kind of late in the day.

Go on, I say.

But there is something more than the flesh, I can tell you that.

I'd like to know what makes you say so.

The many experiences I've had — some could be classified as miracles. I'm sure you've had experiences that are something similar.

Like what?

Well, I don't remember just now, but you come to a point and you know there is something there. You just can't bring it into consciousness.

Do you think you will have a consciousness on the other side?

No, not in this way — not individual consciousness. Too much to hope for.

You seem to have no fear.

No, because the universe is unlimited — no end. No beginning.

So you are on your way to participate in the universe?

Since I have left my wishes to be cremated and scattered in the sea, I'll be back into circulation quickly.

I nod. And I thought of the Native American tribe whose cus-tom it was to lay the body out at the top of the mountain and let the eagles and the vultures come and pick it clean, entering bit by bit

Let Eagles Come

How does part of the world leave the world?

How can wetness leave water?

— RUMI

We never had a chance to talk about immortality, she said.

Let's do, I said.

She had raised her head where she sat crumpled between chair and examining table, eyes closed.

She had raised her head and smiled the Eastern European smile that came of its own will, forcing back the lips to a full set of teeth, as if this flashing smile were a takeover by some irresistible and benevolent force.

I'm dying, she said. I don't want it prolonged.

I just nodded to both assertions and to the others she had not stated.

What about this immortality? I said.

You know it's the universe, the indestructibility of the universe.

I sat quietly and waited for her to continue.

The universe is beyond our understanding. We know some things and then we stop knowing. But there is something more than just what we can know.

What do you *think*?

I think there is something more, but I don't have any opinion.

She paused. Only now did the original smile fade a little. I don't believe in God, she said. So here we are.

I felt her clean honesty cutting into the moment. To face death and not give into what for her would be wishful thinking . . .

There is something more in the human spirit, but, whether we find out or not ... well, the body is perishable.

I'm dying. I don't want it prolonged ...

I remembered her early visits — the smile came then as a shy statement of abstention. She didn't want much done, just to talk about things and share ideas. A little cramping, some gaseous distension — she wasn't sick then. No tests, she said. I have had a long and fruitful life. You should spend your time on more worthwhile projects. That same strong deflection was now present in the way she set aside all but the most sensible and essential.

It will be interesting to exchange some opinions, she says, but it's kind of late in the day.

Go on, I say.

But there is something more than the flesh, I can tell you that.

I'd like to know what makes you say so.

The many experiences I've had — some could be classified as miracles. I'm sure you've had experiences that are something similar.

Like what?

Well, I don't remember just now, but you come to a point and you know there is something there. You just can't bring it into consciousness.

Do you think you will have a consciousness on the other side?

No, not in this way — not individual consciousness. Too much to hope for.

You seem to have no fear.

No, because the universe is unlimited — no end. No beginning.

So you are on your way to participate in the universe?

Since I have left my wishes to be cremated and scattered in the sea, I'll be back into circulation quickly.

I nod. And I thought of the Native American tribe whose custom it was to lay the body out at the top of the mountain and let the eagles and the vultures come and pick it clean, entering bit by bit the digestive tracts of these powerful, graceful, soaring birds, who lifted the dead into themselves, lifting the dead into the heavens. No errands, she said, over there. None of those things people do. We were long past whatever opportunity we may have had to steer this thing off in another direction. This no-tests policy of hers held sway. I'd like to get a CT scan, I had said when she got her left upper abdominal pain. No, she said, I like your idea that this is a spasm of the sphincter of Oddi. That makes sense to me that the little valve at the end of the pancreas should be closing and giving me this pain. And, besides, the pancreatic enzymes you gave me are helping.

But then she started losing weight. I got pushy about the CT scan, but still no dice. This was long after she had asked me if I wanted anything from her home. I don't need anything, I had said. Well, it's time for me to get rid of things. They were good to me, but I don't need them now. I have a collection of boxes, some of them really nice, valuable. My daughters have taken what they want. I like boxes, I said. Instead she brought me an elegantly tattered picture book, which I imagined might be a book of children's stories translated from the original Hungarian. It was called *Homes and Habits of Wild Animals*, published by M. A. Donohue and Company in 1934. Just recently, I had turned the first few pages of this book once again as I was thinking about her rapid dwindling and found, in pencil, in the groping hand of a four or five year old, slanting upward in the right upper margin, one of those first attempts to write a name, someone's own name, probably one of her daughters.

It has some beautiful paintings in it, she had said. It's all about animals. I don't know. Maybe your sons would like it.

I laughed, thinking about the no-errands part. And I tried to imagine what that would be like. She had my curiosity going. What else?

She just shrugged.

And we had nothing more in that moment to say. Even knowing it was close to the last moment and there would be none to follow, even knowing her two daughters, who had come from their homes across the country, were outside the door politely giving up precious time for us to sit together, even knowing as they did so she was telling me things she never said nor *would* say to them, even knowing that we had come face to face with the fear of the unasked important things we would think of later, even so . . . There was nothing more to say.

Then it came to me, the pencil marks, the struggling attempts at making a name in the front of the book, the year 1934. That was her *own name*. It was *her* book. She had given me one of her treasures.

The moment fell in upon itself and opened out again.

Well, then, I said, only one thing left . . .

What's that?

A hug.

She looked confused, then smiled broadly. I reached over to where she was lying against the examining table with her IV in her arm and her clothes wrinkling around her shrinking body, and we hugged. And I felt her, beyond the hump of her spine, her bony ribs folding and unfolding over her last wavering breaths. I felt her in a way I knew I would recognize anywhere.

You believe in something similar? she asked.

Yes. And it occurred to me that I might. It was an answer that became in the moment of its creation not just a courteous gesture.

So that's why I'm not afraid, she said. I'm not looking for reunions with family and things like that. That's why I'm not afraid.

I was standing beside her now, letting her say what was left to say.

It would be interesting to know more, but I know it cannot be conscious. Not this kind of knowledge. Things happen that make us know things. That's all we get.

I had been taking notes furiously, not hiding the fact, even telling her at the beginning to wait until I could find something to write on. Now I looked up from the pad and smiled a mischievous, eyebrow-raising smile and said, You know, of course, I'm going to write about this.

I won't be around to read it.

Yes, but you know it already, more clearly than I will be able to say it.

She just smiled. And we sat there awhile, knowing that she was passing to what she imagined she would pass to, having no resistance to it at all, as if resistance were not even a consideration, riding on the motions of her body, slowing each of its magnificent and meticulous wheels of machinery until it finally stopped, leaving me sitting here with only my writing pad to show for it.

Well, I said finally, I hope you have a good trip.

She laughed. I think I will, she said. Too bad we didn't have a chance to discuss it.

I think we just did, I said.

And she put her head back down, falling into half-sleep, half-dying, everything about her showing a deep fatigue with life.

I put a hand on her shoulder. So let the eagles come, I said.

And she may not have known the story, but she knew the image, for the smile that hit her face stuck there with such force it almost keeled her over. It was, in fact, all I could see as I turned to the door.

You have a nice life with your children and your fine family, she said.

I will, I said, as I turned back to her one last time. We will look for you in the universe.

The Chart in the Window

Please forward to our office as soon as possible:
all medical records pertaining to ——.

So I thought about him for the first time since right after it happened. And what I remembered was his almost embarrassing praise, how he sat in the outer office reading or working on his computer, and if I were late and stopped by to apologize, he would say, Never you mind, Dr. Watts, I'm just so grateful to be seen by one of the best doctors in the world. You just take your time. I'll be here when you're ready.

I didn't take him seriously. I knew he hadn't researched his assessment of my abilities the way the folks do who put together the *Guide to America's Top Physicians*. But he had, for whatever reason, established his confidence and, once locked in, never looked back.

Ours was a complicated arrangement. He had many symptoms and many medications, mostly administered by his psychiatrist and his primary, a holistic MD. My job, if it could be characterized, was to look after his esophagitis. But it was always more than that. I was his sounding board for the aches and pains in his body and those more troublesome ones that occupied his Life. His symptoms were aggravating but not fatal. It was his Life that seemed most problematic.

In this way I came to know a little bit about the train wreck known as his love life. Or maybe just those parts he wanted me to know, parts that indicated his lover had found another lover but was still living in the same house with him because financially they couldn't afford to split. I didn't see how such a thing could go on, but he said it was what it had to be.

Meanwhile, we adjusted his Prilosec, tried him on Propulsid, talked about diet and exercise. He went on Atkins to lose 20 pounds, and I watched as he began to look older somehow, his face flushing with wrinkles the poundage had made less noticeable. He was thinning and aging all in the same gesture.

I've never felt better, he insisted. But if I go off this diet, even one smidge, I start gaining back my weight, and that, well, that's enough to make me unhappy.

You're doing well, I said.

I'm blessed to have such great doctors, he said.

I didn't feel I'd done that much and would have told him so, but I knew he would only argue.

Now this letter I just got wants to know stuff. What do they want to know? Why do they want to know it? What motivates this query? My guess is it's a relative who is requesting, through a lawyer, to see the records. There is no subpoena, so I assume no legal action is pending. Maybe they're just curious. Or maybe they're so saddened that after almost two years they want to know a reason. They could be looking for a way to release their pain, or they could be looking for a way to sue anybody they can catch in the crosshairs. Doctors motor along with a little fear of litigation in the sidecar. To ignore it would be foolish, to pay too much attention would be paranoia. A fishing expedition. Maybe that's what this letter is. How, then, can I trust this little treasury of Robbie to someone I've never met or spoken to or corresponded with save for this cryptic little note?

So I looked for his chart and discovered it had been culled from the office. Must be too old to carry in the files, I thought. No, culled, I remembered, because he is deceased. I looked on the list of charts in storage but couldn't find his name. Finally, I remembered there was a box of charts I'd taken home that got left out in the rain and was drying out slowly in my kitchen. One Sunday I dug in and found him at the bottom of the stack.

So I brought him in, wet and wilting, and placed him on the windowsill in my office looking out over the Golden Gate Bridge where he would collect full sun and restore himself.

But I didn't read him.

Now, I reckon, it's mostly dry. Still, I haven't read it. There will be a difference between what I remember and what I will read, knowing what I know now. The chart itself has changed. There is a different tone going down when reading in reverse.

I wonder if the chart will show or even hint at the level of admiration we had, if it will show the pleasure talking through the pages, the camaraderie.

Out my window, over the view of the chart, a red-tailed hawk circles. A red balloon rises, and it appears to me that the hawk, flying close but without tipping his hand, has just sized up the balloon and with measured circles moves on. He is so near I could almost touch him, almost discover, up close, the coloration at the contrast point between brindle and rust that comes just at the junction of his tail feathers. The hawk is gone. It was windy last night, and the air that got left is sharper than a postcard.

What would Robbie say? I don't need to ask. I can see him throwing his arm in an arc of rejection. Oh, those prying ninnies, he'd say. They're just up to no good. But then, well, he might say, oh, just let them have their fun.

The chart is quiet on this. It sits, unmoving, even though the words inside must be quivering with tension. All that peacefulness and then that last entry. Tucked in to the front page of the chart, his letter.

I get letters all the time. At a glance I can sense the heft or fluff within. This one hit my hand with full awareness, turning around and zeroing in on me like a zoom on a telephoto lens — the postmark, the return address scrawled on the back, the please do not bend or fold written across the left-hand corner as a final urging to preserve image or impulse. My name written with a deliberate, unhurried hand. I tossed the letter lightly to feel it fall in my hand and fine-tuned myself to what was already talking to me from inside.

Tonight, May 6th is the date we have chosen to make our transition from this life. This may shock and sadden many who knew us, but it is an action that was not made lightly. As many of you know we have had struggles for several years now ... we simply ran out of options ... please celebrate our lives as we have ...

And written in the margin in his own hand: *thank you for your wonderful care all these years. Please remember us in the good times as they far outweighed the challenging times. All my love and gratitude ...*

What I remember about that moment was having no feeling at all. Nothing penetrated that whirling void of shock that sucked at me from inside. But even in numbness the body knows how to respond. It's the gesture we make jutting our hand in the air and saying, *Eh,* as if to say, How can what you cannot possibly apprehend tell you what to expect? Then I could feel the beginning of something new. It was absence. He would not be in the outer office reassuring other patients waiting there that all would be well. He would not be bringing his hand-picked flowers. The spot where he was in the world had a hole in it.

No prelude. No finality. It just was. No introduction, no calling card, no rational framework in which to place it. It was as if a part of the landscape out my window had suddenly disappeared and instead of Angel Island, nothing.

Now all this attention to the chart. What does anyone know of this? Yet it comes down to *the chart.* No. *Some*thing comes down to the chart, for both the chart and I agree there is more to this than we know. Nonetheless, there it sits on the windowsill, trying to remember.

It's unavoidable, I conclude. Robbie and I are about to be judged upon what the chart knows but also upon what it might reveal without intending to, the little asides and omissions we do that fit what the relationship has shaped for itself, made of itself. How the conversation works to get done what will not come from pharmacology or technology. In no way is the chart what we were, yet we will be measured by what is there. Such is the intent of eyes that read, angled now with narrow purpose.

Will the chart withstand all this? Will we?

Do not fold or bend. That would be for the photograph with broad smiles on the balcony in sunshine. A postcard from happier times.

So I am sitting in this room with my knowledge of Robbie circulating in my head, and over by the window is the chart with its knowledge, and I know we are different in the way we remember him. And I know that others who can never step inside the doctor-patient relationship as it really was will want to know what the chart knows, and it's possible that through all this the chart has become a third person.

The chart is drying.

The chart is unsticking its pages.

It is getting ready to be read.

Thank You Mr. Nicholson

I am on vacation.

My ear hurts.

Once in a while these buzzy little bacteria that hide under years and years of desquamating ear canal skin rise up and bite me — well, not bite, exactly — start an itch that goes on, if I let it, to become a painful little seep hole in the side of my head.

Not pretty.

Naturally, I did not put the medicine that would make it go away in my dopp kit, packed now under layers of skis, boots, and God knows what my sons have put into those colorful suitcases on wheels they insist upon packing themselves and that show up mysteriously at the front door just before leaving.

We're about to stop for a little shopping — provisions to carry into the deep woods of the condo, something to last us through the long winter nights. This might be an opportunity to get ahold of that potion, that simple formulation, a little drop of steroid and a little antibiotic mixed together in some sterile water, and $45.00 later everything will be alllll rrrrright!

Yes! The supermarket is one of those that comes with a pharmacy — real nice, but they have their rules.

They want my driver's license — okay, address, phone number, California medical license number — yes, indeed. But now they want the actual *medical* license itself. I look at the pharmacist. I suppose you'd like my mother's library card?

She wasn't amused.

I don't have it with me, I say.

Then we can't fill your prescription, she says.

But you know, I say, if I had called you on the phone ...

She's way ahead of me. Yes, she says. I can take your order on the phone. But if you walk into the store and write a prescription, we have to see your medical license.

Let me get this straight, I say. The me on the phone is more reliable than the me in person ...

It's the law, she said.

Of course, I'm sure they mean well, these lawmakers who make laws like that, and I'm sure there's some hardened criminal out there somewhere just waiting for the opportunity to walk into the pharmacy and walk out with some eardrops. But there ought to be one kind of law for the heavy hitters like narcotics and big-time antibiotics and another kind of law for the stuff that wouldn't hurt a flea. Besides, it's a shock to learn I'm more convincing as a doctor on the phone than I am in the flesh.

And I'm looking at her and I'm absolutely certain that none of this quizzical kind of thinking is going to get me anywhere with her, and before long my ear is going to turn into a sump.

And right here in the middle of this moment I remember Jack Nicholson as Robert Dupea in *Five Easy Pieces*, that scene where he's trying to order an omelet and toast but the waitress won't give him a side of toast. So he figures out a way: he'll get his toast if he orders a chicken salad sandwich, hold the butter, hold the lettuce, hold the mayonnaise, and then he says, *Now all you have to do is hold the chicken, bring me the toast, give me a check for a chicken salad sandwich, and you haven't broken any rules.*

I look down at the counter. There, looking like a miniature billboard sitting in its little billboard rack is a stack of the pharmacist's business cards. I take one. I look back up at her. Perhaps if I were more like Robert Dupea I'd have the fiery streak that would make me pull out my cell phone right then and there and call her up, face to face. But then he got thrown out of the restaurant for stunts like that and never did get his omelet and toast.

I walk a few aisles away into the ladies cosmetics. I can still see the pharmacist when someone answers my call.

Hello, is this the pharmacist?

No, let me get her. And she puts me on hold.

Presently, someone calls to the person who was just standing in front of me, and she turns to answer the phone.

Hello, she says. This is the pharmacist.

Good, I say. This is Dr. Watts.

And it may be my imagination, but I could swear that the look in her eyes could melt nails.

Go ahead, she says.

I'd like to order a small bottle of Cortisporin.

Sig?

qtts ii bid prn.

Will generics do?

Sure.

Do we have you on computer?

No, I don't think so.

Let me get your address.

I give it.

Your telephone number.

I give it.

Your California license number.

I give it.

Okay, she says, it'll be ready in about fifteen minutes.

Swell, I say, and you see, we haven't broken any rules.

Talking about Christmas

You have a different philosophy than I do, she said. And though by saying that she made me pause and think about it for a minute, she did not change my mind.

It was the doctor speaking, my mother's doctor, and we were having a disagreement. I had assumed that when she went to see my mother in the nursing home the day before and found the signs of bronchitis or perhaps pneumonia, those signs I had intuited over the phone by talking to my mother and to her helpers, the doctor would put her in the hospital.

The next day my mother was still in the nursing home, and no antibiotics had been ordered.

That's when I called.

It was almost Thanksgiving, and, starting the week before, I had been thinking about my mother's love for Christmas and how she always began months before making and hiding gifts, how every ornament on the tree had a story behind it — perhaps some interesting tidbit about the person who gave it to us or how it hung every Christmas on her mother's tree in Laredo or the time we found it in the antique store — how she would write a poem or compose a little song for me and my brother and then eventually in later years for her grandchildren, an attempt, perhaps, to reach over the distance placed by time and geography and prickly daughters-in-law, and how I remembered as a child in her house, in that brief and luminous season, how all my worries disappeared . . .

So when the return call came, it was from this doctor I'd never met, saying, Your mother's not doing well.

I know, I said. The attendant told me she was feverish and having difficulty breathing. Since you were scheduled to see her in the next half-hour I guess I kind of assumed she was as good as in the hospital.

And I was thinking that now I had found myself smack dab in the middle of a health-care discussion not unlike those I'd had many times before, only this time not as the doctor but as family.

I'm not sure what I can do for her, the doctor was saying. I'd have to restrain her just to keep her from pulling off her oxygen. Besides, it looks like an aspiration pneumonia, which means her Alzheimer's is messing up her swallowing mechanism. If she does pull through, she probably won't be able to nourish herself.

And I thought to myself, That's what we do. What you've just described *is* the practice of medicine — the cleverness with which we design treatment even in the face of difficulty. Even so, the doctor had made her point. As she did so the feeling spread through me that she had written my mother off. I'd never had that feeling before, and it was shockingly strange. Mother was fading, and here we were negotiating not the method of her care but her manner of dying.

We were both silent awhile, listening to our silences rise together in the telephone lines as if they should be telling us something.

I was trying to decide if the doctor's reluctance was appropriate or harsh. And I could feel the friction of my divided selves rubbing together, my doctor self and my son self. One side was trying to contain those swirling emotions, and the other, not wanting to dampen them, believed they might have arisen from some truth we'd overlooked.

It had to be played out.

It's her first episode, I said. With a little help she might recover.

The doctor sighed, which signaled to me she thought the hospitalization would be more for my benefit than my mother's. She could be right. But her coolness animated me, and I pressed on.

Restrain her for a while, I said. Give her fluids. Who knows, she could recover and do all right for weeks, even months.

The doctor in me was listening and thinking about what I'd just said. Maybe the important thing was not that it was my *mother's* first episode but that it was *mine*.

I was asking myself questions. Was I being too aggressive? Was I expecting more from my mother than from one of my own patients?

No. If Mother suffered pain or if her life was paralyzed by fear or anxiety, it might be different. But she kisses the hands of everyone who comes in her room, saying, I love you. Do you have to go away?

Your philosophy is different from mine, she said.

And it occurred to me that my mother, even in her rational poverty, still had the gift to bless and to make people smile. Maybe intelligence is overrated as the cardinal sign of a successful state of being.

You don't know her, I said. She's a great lady.

And as I said this two parts of me were listening, one proud to say what I had said and standing behind it, the other a little embarrassed to be expressing what almost everyone feels about their mother.

Well, as it turned out, the doctor caved in and admitted my mother to the hospital, started fluids, IV antibiotics, oxygen. Mother was going to be okay for a while. It felt right.

As I left to go to the airport my wife asked what I was going to say to my mother. In my mind was the visit with her last spring in which there were moments she couldn't even hold on to my name. How best to celebrate the part of her that still remained?

Well, I said, I think we'll talk about Christmas.

And she *did* remember my name, and we *did* talk about Christmas, as if the conversation we had been having all our lives had never been interrupted, not by time or distance or the cruel penalties of aging. And there were moments when she looked as sprightly as she had when she was making and hiding presents for "my wonderful boys." And then suddenly she would tire and say, I think I'll sleep now, David. And then I'd say, Okay, and drift back to my motel. It was good. Very good. I wouldn't have missed it for anything.

I went back to California. She was discharged from the hospital. It was the last time I saw my mother.

She made it through Christmas, which was a simple affair: a few relatives stopping by the nursing home, some flowers, a jar of peanuts, my telephone call from San Francisco through which I marched my not-so-recently-new wife and two new boys, whom she would occasionally confuse with my other family and have to be reminded whom she was talking to, and then to say, Oh, David, I'm sorry. I just don't seem to have the energy to do the things I used to do for Christmas. You remember, don't you? Weren't those wonderful times we had together? I'm so tired. Will you call again?

Then one day not long after, deep in winter, just after the start of the new year, I got the call I had been expecting but trying hard not to. This time the doctor was calling from the hospital. I'm sorry, David, she said. Your mother is gone.

It was early morning in California, two hours after the same early morning in Texas, and the sun was just lighting the trees over the skylight above our bed. My wife reached over and hugged me. I didn't know to expect that, and it broke me open.

When the call came he would say the words
he had rehearsed but would not remember

words somehow that still needed
to be spoken . . . and he recognized

how empty, and at the same time how necessary,
words can be,

as the first light of the first day without his mother
crept into the trees . . .

Silence Knows the
Right Questions

A woman came to see me with headaches. Maybe it was Georgina. She'd had them a long time, she said, ten years maybe, and had tried all sorts of medications, seen all sorts of doctors, suffered all sorts of side effects at the hands of well-intended but off-the-mark interventions, but without relief. She had become so disgusted with the whole damn mess she'd just given up. She'd told her friend she'd gotten more misery than help, and she was just learning the hell to live with it.

Her friend said, You have to go see Dr. Watts.

Not another doctor, she said.

Before you give up, see Dr. Watts.

So now she sits across the desk from me, and something about her the instant she walked in the room told me to keep my damn mouth shut.

So I do.

And she begins.

And she tells me the history of her illness in the manner she has been taught, in the manner learned from seeing all those doctors, learning to speak the academic language of clinicians and the expectations placed upon it: how long it has been going on, how each headache begins, what helps, what doesn't, where the pain is, what the pain feels like, what the pain level is on a scale of 10, the precipitating factors . . .

They say the average time it takes a doctor to interrupt a patient as she is trying to tell her story is about thirteen seconds. I believe it. They've studied that somewhere, and I remember it now. Doctors are trained to do that. Medical schools want the doctor to make the patient's history conform to the logical flow of reasoning, of explication, of the detective-like progression of science that makes its calculated and measured steps toward a logical conclusion. The trouble with illness is that it's only logical in the abstract, not in the human. Mixed with the human personality, illness is often irrational.

Something about her said, Let her be. Discovery is at her lead. So "It" will have to take us where it wants.

So she talks.

And she talks.

And then she stops.

She's been talking for about five minutes now, talking as if she were delivering a recitation of some sort, a poem memorized for the third-grade teacher who demands it from her reluctant pupils, some tale pressed into her memory and from which she is now detached, careless as she moves through it while by its own dull energy — surely not hers — it drones and meanders . . . And I can see she is expecting some dry response, the chemical solution that does not work scribbled on a little piece of paper . . .

She is silent now. Weary.

And the problem rests upon the desk between us, not speaking. But the problem has not been opened. It is a closed box, and I cannot see the latch.

Silence.

I know there has to be a right question, *but I don't know what it is.*

Perhaps in disappointment in the face of the abject dullness of her new physician, she seems almost dreamy, her eyes drifting off to the side.

I have learned only a few things, but I know that there are times when more gets done in silence than in speaking. The road signs have been removed. I let the silence run, thirty seconds, maybe even a minute . . . Silence knows the right questions.

Then she sort of startles, as if waking. You know, she says at last, brushing an invisible tuft of lint from her skirt, something happened to me last week that I do not understand.

I gesture with my hand for her to continue, unwilling to break the spell.

She is looking down as she speaks. Maybe she didn't see me gesture. Still, she rises to continue in the river of thought.

I was going to visit my accountant on the twenty-fifth floor of the Bank of America Building — it's something I do every month — and I realized for the first time in my life . . . and she pauses here as if testing the words she is about to say . . . then presses forward . . . I suddenly realized that I . . . did not want to be in the same elevator with my husband.

Then she turns and looks straight at me, fixing me with her hard, demanding eyes, and says, What do you think that means?

Now this is a dangerous moment.

I have known this woman exactly six and a half minutes, and I have not earned the right, even though I know, even though almost any third person listening to her tale would know, at least some piece of the answer, I have not earned the right to tell her what to do with her life.

I say, I don't know what it means. I'm not sure. But I do know it's really important.

So she and I sit with this new important thing in the room, both of us beginning to feel its shape and its texture.

Do me a favor, I said. Think about this awhile and then come back and see me.

So she went away.

And then she came back.

Two weeks had passed. And in that short period of time she had stored her furniture, moved out, and started divorce proceedings.

Wow! I said.

Wow! she said. I guess I've needed to do that for a long, long time.

And we sat in the wow of that moment, not wanting to either embellish or detract from the power that comes from finding something hidden so long.

You found this, she said.

No. I didn't even know where to look.

I think you did.

I think you needed a place where it was possible to hear yourself talk. When it was quiet enough for that timid voice, you heard the answer.

Maybe, she said.

Something like that, I said.

And you know what? she said.

What?

Don't you know?

I stuck by my silence. It had served me well.

She was looking at me as if I had forgotten something so simple, so elemental, so obvious.

My headaches are gone, she said.

One Cancer Cell

What do you do with one cancer cell?

Jonathan Katchaturian is sitting on the edge of the endoscopy table for his repeat procedure, the one that wouldn't have been done this early but for the fact that the pathology report on his esophageal biopsy last month said "one cancer cell."

Then there was a comment.

We don't know, it said, *whether this cell belongs to this biopsy or if it "floated on."*

Floated on. I imagined a cancer cell somehow misplaced in the staining bath of hematoxylin and eosin, floating disoriented there without a country, detached from some faraway superpower that passed through the region and left behind something to be remembered by, a sentry, a derelict foot soldier waiting for some unsuspecting, innocent sliver of someone else's tissue to wander by and provide a resting place. Does it know the consternation it caused by this little game?

The report went on.

There is nothing in the microanatomy of the biopsy specimen to suggest malignancy or even premalignancy. Yet this cell is definitely malignant.

So Jonathan is back. For one thing, I wanted to make sure this cell didn't float in from his *own* tissue, some factory of malevolence in a nearby region that has sloughed a single cell like a warning flare onto the playing field.

And I know we make cancer cells all the time, and they are, for the most part, snarfed up by our killer cells, a necessary defense system we have evolved to make over the missteps we fumble into from time to time. Was this one of those?

You know how much I love this procedure, he says.

Me too. And I raise one eyebrow.

We tease each other, but we both know we can't let the cancer issue go unattended even if it is just one cell. So we are decided. And here we go.

So what have I told him?

Well. I've said I'm not very worried, which is true. But what do I know? I know cancer didn't get the moniker "malignant" for accomplishments in good behavior. Does he have cancer if he has one cell? What do I *really* know?

For one, I know that that little cancer cell was out of place. There was nothing in the endoscopy to suggest a cancer or anything remotely looking like a cancer. And I know that cells do sometimes drift in the staining bath of the pathology lab and "metastasize" to the next available microscopic slide. But cancer is no small thing to reckon with. Beyond all that I don't know a damn thing. And that's where the rub comes in.

So we act like this is routine, knowing we are acting and knowing we both feel the one little stitch in our sides that starts with the letter *c*. Acting sometimes is as good as the real thing. Maybe better.

There is a difference and a similarity in the way Jonathan and I think about this little cancer cell. My thinking is shaped by percentages, by the odds that this little bugger will be attached to some greater, life-threatening process, and I know from my training that that scenario is not likely. His thinking is based on the emotional response to the concept of something growing that cannot be stopped and the urgency one feels to generate action without possibility of delay. The thing about it is this: I feel every emotion he feels, but my job is to override with perspective. Therefore, I act coolish on the outside and at the same time tend to the things we both worry about on the inside. I am trying to balance the emotional with the rational. That's not always a successful project.

As the endoscope arrives at its target I scrutinize the region in question. I scour the area like a sleuth after reticent clues. I biopsy the tissue maybe ten times. The tissue looks normal. I biopsy it anyway. I examine every suspect in the region, the fundus, the angulus, the pylorus, and the slinky duodenum.

We did our job, I say to him afterward. There was nothing there.

He asks the repeat question I know he will ask because in stressful times the brain is a little slow to pick up the corrective concepts. I answer him as many times as he asks.

Now to wait for the path report. Times like these the clock ticks audibly, and the music from *Who Wants to Be a Millionaire* comes to mind.

In four days it came: Nothing. Zilch. Zoley. Zero.

Now what?

Well, at least it's what we expected, I tell him. And the news is good. That little floater may be just about done as an issue, but it's not done with our consciousness just yet.

Jonathan goes home assured.

I go home assured. Mostly. One of the differences between us is that it is my duty to reassure. And I have done that. And with genuine conviction, because I do believe the outcome is good and belief is what drives us to confidence. But that leaves me with the doubt to deal with. Better me than him, I say. And here's how I do it.

We plan endoscopies every six months for two years. I will let him subscribe to the belief that all is well, while I make sure nothing happens on my watch. Maybe I'm treating myself, but if nothing comes of this by the time we have done the ritual maybe three or four times — whatever satisfies the soul at this point — we will call it quits. We both agree on that. What has happened is that the ritual, like Unguentine, has absorbed the caustic burn of doubt. We can both set aside worry, knowing there is a reasonable mechanism in place to watch the store.

And that's what we do. We put it out of our minds, resting the urge to become frightened directly upon the shoulders of surveillance, which have been structured to bear this load, matching not the risk of that one cancer cell but the horror that came with it to the action we have chosen.

Anathema

You're going to love this one, she says and backs out of the room.

I flash briefly on all the problem children in my practice, but they fade quickly from my mind, for I know by the tone of her voice she is talking about the cranky problem, the thorn-in-the-side problem, the anathema ... *the insurance company*.

Perhaps she's remembering the rare times I have raised my voice on the phone or had the audacity to ask the insurance company doctor where he went to medical school or if he'd actually seen a patient since the Korean War. By all this I'm pretty sure of the subject, only not, just yet, the issue.

Wait a second, I say.

We've had this one before, she says from the hall, still stepping backward.

Had what?

There is a new chart on the corner of my desk next to the place where she was just standing but has left. I can almost see it breathing.

It's a Remicade denial, she says as she slips around the corner into her office and shuts the door.

Remicade is a high-stakes game that the insurance companies hate because it is a medicine that is both a lifesaver — which means they have a hard time justifying why they should turn down payment for it — and it's as expensive as hell. Just the exact combination that gets their goat.

Remicade is a sophisticated treatment for autoimmune disorders, diseases in which the body fights against itself, some misadventure of mistaken identity — a glitch in the immune system that allows antibodies like wayward missiles to attack the home turf. Friendly fire, so to speak.

This arrangement of confusion is a costly one, for it results in diseases like psoriasis, rheumatoid arthritis, and in the field of gastroenterology — ulcerative colitis and Crohn's disease.

These poor people have the misfortune of suffering what might be likened to arthritis of the bowel and, in some cases, go without a satisfactory treatment anywhere on the planet. By the time they get to Remicade they have usually failed antibiotics, aspirin compounds, steroids, and even the scary immunosuppressives. Then once they get on Remicade — miracle of miracles — most of them suddenly get better.

Jonna, the patient in question, used to suffer pain and diarrhea so bad she couldn't work to support her children and was always moody and miserable. Now all that's history, and she's showing up for her Remicade infusions, driving sixty miles in heavy traffic, puffing and panting like it was a privilege just to be here.

Well, I knew the insurance company couldn't find a way to refuse the treatment on the grounds that it didn't work, so it has to come down to a technicality. We know this.

The chart is conspicuous on the corner of my desk. I laugh and then go and find my administrator. So what is it this time?

It's the weight, she says.

Weight?

Yeah, we reported it in pounds and they want it in kilos.

Let me get this straight. They refused the whole reimbursement . . . what is it? About five thousand dollars?

Six . . .

. . . because the weight was in pounds not kilos.

Right.

They can't divide by 2.2?

She just looks at me.

Don't answer that, I say. So they turned down all our expenses.
Six thousand dollars' worth.

Figures.

You're going to have to talk to them this time.

I smile an ironic smile. It *was* kind of funny. I have to stop seeing patients — stamping out disease, as my mentor used to call it — to go talk to some clerk somewhere in Iowa or maybe India who has refused to authorize payment due in full because we gave them an *accurate* number in *inaccurate* units. Ah, technicalities, the power they have to preside over good medicine.

So, after keeping Lorna on hold for forty-five minutes — during which time she kept her ear open to the tinny musaq-like annoyance while I go back to Mrs. Laudebaum in the examining room — a voice comes on the line. This is a dangerous moment. You have to be real quick and real loud because if they don't hear a response instantly, they'll hang up, and you'll have to start all over again at the end of the queue.

They're on the line, Lorna says, and I stop taking a blood pressure, excuse myself, and come to the phone.

You owe me six thousand dollars, I said.

You didn't fill out the form right, she said.

Okay. But if you divide 144 by 2.2 you get . . . um . . . 65.5 kilos.

You have to put it on the form.

It's right in front of you. Why don't you do it?

You have to.

If I put it on the form and send it back to you, it will take another three months before we can have this conversation about some other trumped-up technicality.

It's the only way, she said.

Now, I knew the results of the next interchange in advance, but, being miffed by the principle of it all, I couldn't resist.

You mean you're going to withhold a valuable treatment for a sick patient on the basis of a technicality.

We're not withholding the treatment, we're just refusing to pay for it.

Same difference.

What?

You know very well the patient can't afford this out of pocket. That's why she bought insurance in the first place.

Silence.

If you withhold six thousand dollars, it's the same as denying treatment.

Silence.

And now that I look at the record I see that you haven't paid us for the treatment before this one either. I'm not a bank. Not to mention that this little trick means you can keep the money you owe me and collect interest on it. Making money on my money. I should charge *you* interest for late payment.

We can't do that.

Do you charge interest for late payments on your premiums?

Well, yes.

Another thing. I can't walk into Macy's and walk out with a sport jacket without paying for it on the spot. My services have been rendered just as surely as Macy's rendered me the sport jacket. How can you get away with this?

You have to do the paperwork right.

Yeah, yeah. You have to do your paperwork. You have to do your paperwork.

So this has turned out exactly as I expected. No response to the logical appeal, no response to the compassionate appeal. This is how they make their money. I guess I'll have to play my trump card.

What is your name? I ask.

There was a pause during which I imagined I could hear the electrons of her brain cursing and spitting. And then, reluctantly, and only because she knew she had to, she gave it.

Do you realize, Donna (we'll call her), that because you have refused to pay the bill, money that you already owe me, you may compromise the health of this patient?

We're not doing that.

Ah, but you are. My office cannot afford to carry such large sums of money outstanding for months and months at a time while you wait around to decide if and when to pay it.

No answer.

Look, I *bought* the Remicade with my own money and *paid* the nurse to come and start the IV, give the premedications, and supervise the infusion. This is expensive stuff, and payment is overdue. Now you've enlarged my debt on a technicality. You've got all the information you need.

No answer.

There came a moment in which I felt a little sorry for the clerk, this clerk who is doing exactly what she is trained to do by the hard-line capitalists in the company. But as a human in the system she could have put the number in as I gave it to her and bypassed another long roundabout for my patient. She has personal responsibility for her actions. Not since the Nuremberg trials has anyone been able to get away with saying, *I was just following orders.* My moment of sympathy for her passed as quickly as it came. My allegiance is with Jonna, who's going to start fading if she doesn't get her Remicade — she'll get her diarrhea back, she'll start feeling puny and weary . . . We'll lose the progress we've made. It's about her comfort, her welfare, her children . . .

So here goes.

Listen, Donna, I say. Suppose I hold you *personally* responsible for the health of this woman. Suppose I take the position that because you wouldn't calculate the number you wanted from the number we gave you or even take the correct number over the phone, thus correcting the paperwork, you are preventing a critical treatment to a sick woman. What do you suppose any reasonable person would think of that?

No answer.

I'll tell you what. You go ahead and refuse treatment, and then, if anything bad happens to my patient, if she gets sick or goes to the hospital or has to have surgery, I'm going to give her your name and the name of the best damn lawyer I know.

Silence.

I think that's the end of my little message, I say and hang up the phone.

Next day the fax comes.

We're approved! my assistant says.

By now I have forgotten all about this. Despite the sharp peak of acrimony, these interactions with insurance companies are so common as to be salt underfoot.

Remicade. Remicade! she says.

Oh yeah. Oh yeah, I say. Good.

We take a deep breath.

And then we go back to what we were doing.

Telling the Truth in the Realm of Truth

Do you know what he told me?

Already I had the picture: my patient sitting in the office of the Second Opinion Doctor, listening with all her being to what he had to say. Patients always get a different opinion there, at the Second Opinion Doctor, even if it's not *much* different. That's part of the psychology of second opinions and why they work.

So here I am, she says, thinking that we've been doing everything we were supposed to be doing, and he blew me out of the water.

I knew she was excitable, questioning, nervous, among my patients the one who is most involved at every level of decision making. I also knew she had a low threshold both for excitability and for pain. She has Crohn's disease or colitis, it's hard to tell, one of those in-between bowel diseases that catapults its way back and forth between diagnoses. Bottom line: pain and sometimes diarrhea. But always pain. She has to take a little narcotic most days just to get by.

And yet the exams of the bowel are often unimpressive. Somehow there is a little disconnect between symptoms and the magnitude of disease. Oh yes, there has been the occasional patch of inflammation, but mostly, at least at the times we held the spotlight to it, the colon has looked okay. Biopsies okay. Until, that is, that one fateful time when *dysplasia* showed its face.

The word *dysplasia* strikes terror, terror in both of us — for me the sudden shock that on my watch one of my patients is going down the road to cancer, for her . . . well . . .

Dysplasia!!! she shrieked in the moment when I first told her. Oh my god, I've heard that word and I hate it already. What does it mean?

So I start with the analogy of the Pap smear: low-grade aberration is dysplasia, high-grade, cancer. That's a system that works, I say, because there is a definable and predictable gradation that calls out increasingly louder alarm signals the higher you go up the ladder. It's reliable, like Smokey the Bear's fire warnings.

Now I look her in the eye. But it's not the same in the colon, I say. They can tell cancer . . . and normal . . . but not as much certainty at the stages between the two.

You haven't answered my question.

I'm setting the stage. The cell that is dysplastic is thinking about becoming a cancer.

Thinking about?

Thinking about — not cancer, not normal. Problem is, in the colon nobody knows the direct connection between the two or how long it takes.

What do we do? What do we do? I can't stand this kind of indecision. All this is fine, but what are we going to do about it?

I considered how to say the next part. Straight out would be best. Some people recommend taking out the colon, I said.

The whole colon?

All of it.

Why? That doesn't make sense.

Well, if you believe that once dysplasia happens in one part of the colon, it is happening or about to happen in other parts of the colon, and if you believe that dysplasia leads directly to cancer without passing Go, then one sure way to avoid the problem is to take out the whole colon.

Is that the way it works?

My opinion is that it is unclear. And I also believe you can't even be sure of the condition of dysplasia on one sample. It might be distorted somehow. Accidents happen in the pathology lab. Readers of samples vary from day to day. There are variables. It's kind of like saying, "One swallow does not a spring make."

Oh great!

A conservative path, I paused as I said this, is to go back in and check for dysplasia again. And if it's not there, check again every few weeks or months for a while. But if you get dysplasia one more time, and the pathologists say it's likely precancerous . . . well, I'd probably recommend surgery.

And if not?

If not, you can keep on going.

Going how?

Checking periodically.

What good is that?

Well, it might save your colon. Because if we don't find dysplasia or something else alarming, we'll assume it was a fluke.

Does that happen?

Everything happens. Dysplastic cells can revert back to normal or die or disappear. I found a cancer cell once — *one* cancer cell — one single cell on a biopsy of the esophagus from one of my patients. I didn't believe it, so we went back several times and never found it again. He's still alive and well fifteen years later — *with* his esophagus.

But what I want to know is, is it safe to go this way.

I know it may be frustrating, but no one knows for sure. Not at the level of one hundred percent, anyway. But if you're watching it frequently . . .

What are you watching for?

Behavior.

Cells have behavior?

You bet.

I knew that. I knew that. So what are you saying?

It's a reasonable, not an overly dramatic solution to the problem.

So the story is, we went with that. And three colonoscopies later . . . no dysplasia.

But her symptoms of pain and diarrhea came back, roaring back, and they didn't respond to any of my medicines, not steroids, not immunosuppressives, anti-inflammatories, the works. Not even Remicade. So she started worrying to the tune of "something bad must be going on in there."

I'm pretty confident it's still okay, I said, especially since you've got irritable bowel syndrome too, and then there's that low threshold thing.

She raised her eyebrows.

Yes, I know, I said. But this is no time to patronize you or the situation at hand. You feel everything that goes on in your bowel. You're *wired* that way.

And I was thinking about the opposite end of the spectrum, how my medical student patient wasn't wired that way at all. She, age twenty-seven, had had fifteen years of abdominal pain, starting with the onset of her menstrual period at age twelve, ending up as endometriosis. She had lived so long with pain she almost didn't know it was there. Examining her, pushing my hand into her lower abdomen, I asked if it was painful. She had to recall the incident that just that second passed us by to decide if she had pain or not, the disconnect was that strong.

The student just assumed that pain was part of life, even though she had pain with sex, pain with bowel movements, and pain at unpredictable times that awakened her at night. She couldn't place her legs flat on the table. I was very impressed. She had suffered so sweetly that she almost cried when she finally found someone who would pay attention to her pain.

I turned back to the opposite situation. I think, just to be safe, I said, we should get a CT scan of the abdomen — that'll help us be sure there are no surprises there — and then send you off for a second opinion. I know a GI guy who specializes in inflammatory bowel diseases.

You're suggesting a second opinion?

Sure. Difficult or complex situations benefit from one more brain in the think tank. Besides, it's another way to check against the possibility of something missed.

So she saw the Second Opinion Guy, and then she called me up, freaking out.

Do you know what he said? She was practically screaming on the phone. He said I should have had my colon out the very minute we first found dysplasia, and if it was him he would have taken it out right away. Excuse me for saying so but he scared the *shit* out of me.

It took a beat or two for the details to come back under my command. As I was booting up my brain-computer my first worry was we hadn't done proper surveillance. Or done it often enough. Or that there was some new study I was not aware of that prompted this urgent response. As is my habit, my first flash was that the conflicting opinion was correct.

No. Wait a minute. The discussions, the colonoscopies without finding dysplasia were slowly coming back to me. There was very little chance we'd missed cancer or even precancer.

Well, that *is* one of the reigning opinions, I said. But I think we talked about that.

Yes. Or *maybe* we did. I can't remember. But here I am thinking I'm doing what I am supposed to do, doing what *you told me to do*, and now I'm really scared we've let this go to a point that something really bad is about to happen.

I still think we're okay.

Then why did he say that?

Well, I guess he believes it.

But that's directly contrary to what you said. How can that be?

It's extreme, I said, but not that different. The extreme of what we also talked about but decided not to do.

But he was adamant. He spoke with urgency, like I was being remiss for running around with this colon still in me.

It was hard for me to represent these two opinions and how they could be part of the same truth.

Maybe he overspoke, I offered.

Scary. And now I'm not so sure we've done the right thing.

And now we must consider he's right. But he probably didn't know whom he was talking to.

What do you mean?

How you might be affected by his tone of voice, the insistency, the strong approach.

Well, no, I just met him, and suddenly he's practically scream-ing at me.

What he doesn't know, probably, is the effect that will have, I mean on you in particular. That's why I say he didn't know who . . .

No. And I know I'm emotional. But I haven't been able to sleep since he talked to me.

What does he want to do?

He wants to do a colonoscopy.

So fine, I said. Good idea. That's what I'd say about now.

So should I do that?

Absolutely.

Should he do it?

Why not?

And he talked to you, didn't he? I mean, I think he left me in the room and called you up.

Yup, he called me up.

Yeah, I figured that. You know, I have to say that after the conversation with you he came back in the room and was much less animated about it all.

Maybe he understood my point better. Still, it looks like he shook your cage.

Well, I'd say so.

So we agreed to do what the Second Opinion Guy said, to the letter. And then we'd see where we landed. And then one day I ran into the Second Opinion Guy, so I asked him what's up. He'd scheduled her for a colonoscopy, or thought he had, but not for some time yet. Not sure of the date. It seemed the suddenly urgent-urgent had become suddenly not-so-urgent.

It was a long time before I heard anything. Then I got a call from my patient asking for the results of the colonoscopy. I didn't know it had been done, so I went online to the data bank and pulled it down. Normal colonoscopy. Normal biopsy. No dysplasia in any of the four areas biopsied. Not even inflammation.

I told her.

Wow!

Feel better?

Yeah, but I'm really upset.

Why?

Yeah, I went all this time thinking I was dying or something, and it was really okay all along. I'm pissed.

Don't be. Be ecstatic.

Yeah, but to frighten me that way. Why do doctors do that? I had a friend who had a little cut on his lip, and his dentist recoiled in horror, saying he had to get that cancer right off of there. Turned out to be nothing.

Probably thought he was doing a good deed.

I've been thinking about writing to the medical school where he went and asking them why they don't teach doctors how to talk to patients. To be so cocksure and to be so wrong. Scared me half to death.

Remember, he was telling the truth as he saw it.

No, I don't agree. Doctors are not supposed to just tell information. They are supposed to put it into context.

That's the fine tuning, I said.

What do you mean?

Well, here's what I think. He and I both told the truth as we saw it. There were differences in both substance and context. The big difference was that because he stated his version strongly, it frightened you. Then you and he ended up with different ideas about the meaning of what he said. He may have said the truth, but he didn't say the truth into your understanding.

What do you mean?

To speak the truth into the *realm* of truth you sometimes have to say it differently from the way you understand it. Look, the first job of telling the truth is to know what the truth really is. That's a hard job. Truth at its best is mutable. Its parts are constantly changing, and what you see depends on how it is viewed and by whom it is viewed. The second job is to tell what you understand in a manner that the person listening, with all her differences in frame of reference, background understanding, emotional constructs that inform how she sees and hears things . . . taking all that into consideration . . . make sure she comes away with an understanding similar to yours.

You're saying we didn't hear the same.

You didn't hear the same. But I'm also saying he didn't say it in your language. A doctor is supposed to share not just truth but wisdom, which, if you will, is a commentary on the truth. But you haven't shared truth *or* wisdom if you haven't shared it into the perceptual framework of your listener.

You make it sound mutable.

This episode, worse suddenly, caused us to look again at the signals to see if some different clarity might emerge: X-ray the abdomen, looking for the gaseous telltale signs of partial bowel obstruction, get serum enzymes that might suggest a pancreatitis attack, examine the abdomen, in this case, finding a greater amount of tenderness in the epigastrium, that little inverted V-shaped space at the base of the sternum where the stomach lies, and welcome that, just any aberration, to give us a slightly new take on the plane crash. And welcome the new buzzword: gastric outlet obstruction.

So I asked her, How long after she ate did the pain worsen?

Almost immediately.

Is there bloating?

Absolutely.

Did it take a long time to ease off?

Yes.

Was all that connected to the nausea?

Indeed.

And I'm thinking, almost with a kind of bizarre excitement, that it is always a good thing to have a theory, some thin line to hang all this weighty laundry on, something that even though it does not lead to resolution will give a target to throw a few mudballs of blame at. Somebody has to take shit for all this misery. Why not gastric outlet obstruction?

Well, I have to say that I never felt better than after that endo-... that doctor... what was his name? Tum... Tee...

Talkington?

Ah, Talkington. Yeah, he dilated something in me, and I felt for days.

This theory we'd been piecing out of these little signals has something better to do than sitting around doing nothing, it made sense, sort of. That, plus high motivation to do something, makes doing something a slam dunk.

Not only that, you *create* the truth for the benefit of your listener. Each listener. In that way our understandings match. If he failed you, that's the place.

I'm still going to write to his medical school.

You're steamed. But don't blame him. Just ask them to teach their medical students how to transfer truth across the doctor-patient divide. That'll keep them busy.

So I shouldn't kill the medical school?

And don't kill the doctor either. If he can't put the truth into your realm of truth, then try to understand it in his.

That shouldn't be my job.

Well, you've got that right.

So we've since waltzed along, she and I, constraints relaxed, turbulence set aside, though I still keep thinking about that one dysplastic biopsy, and there in a little mailbox right beside it, my best approximation of the translating machinery I need to keep her on the same page I'm on. Which means I wasn't going to mention it again for a long time, keeping vigilance in my own way, shielding my concerns, letting small signals escape through to drip like ink drops in a pool of water, spreading color and particles and ideas and perspective that keep us as close as we can possibly be to what we need to know.

Ghosts in the Machine

You don't know what size you'd need?

Yeah. Fourteen.

Fourteen?

Yeah.

The nurse pulls out the number 14 balloon dilator, which will soon descend through the technical channel, the benevolent channel, the pathway through the endoscope to somewhere in the small bowel — that same somewhere we plan to dilate.

Or not. By now I have pulled up the old endo report, the one from 1999, when the doctor dilated her before — after which she *never felt so good.*

Only he didn't. Didn't dilate. I see it here. There is no mention of dilation anywhere in the report, no balloons, no stricture, none of it.

We have been a long time coming here, a long time with pain, bloating, nausea, these malicious maladies that take away the life force, zones of disability that seem to creep in without explanation or at best a poor one. Living with symptoms is bad enough; living with symptoms *and* uncertainty is murderous.

There have been surgeries in the past, lots of them, ample opportunity for the violin strings of healing to go awry and weave adhesions, the little strangulators of the belly cavity. All those insults that turn the abdomen into a veritable glue pot — not the kind of pond to go into for a fishing expedition.

So we've kept our surgical distance. Do no harm. The monster you know is better than the one you create — all that jazz.

I really don't like pain, she says.

The nurse responds. Nobody likes pain, she says.

I'm really in to starting a new career, she says. I've got the people writing now — it works wonders for their pain. Three more referrals this week, one of them a Franciscan priest who memorizes poetry. It's mesmerizing.

And I'm thinking, This is an example of how we turn our sorrows into something worthwhile. She, a psychologist, has made support group for patients with chronic pain. Who better to l such an enterprise? Who more qualified?

I'm going to write an article, she says.

Really? For who?

We belong to the Catholic Church, and they want to kn the hell we are doing that works.

Speaking of works, I say, how about a little more joy ju we do this thing?

You know, she says, I think I'm going to keep you.

That's because you have Demerol in your veins.

No, she says, it's because I've got *brains* in my he

I do not shake off the compliment. Secretly, I admiration is the one sure thing in this fragile r leads us to pathways, well, maybe small hints of can take through this big thicket we're in. No magic wands. She has pain that would drive m came across it once in our lifetimes, much Everything she eats is sure to increase the bl ing the handle on the winch that wraps he windlass and squeezes from her all mem without pain. Years like this. Frequent vi we tinker with the small things of life: sr ones, just the right amount of fiber that plug her up, enzymes to help what we breaking down to speed up the dig logic, but it's more than a bit myste

So now we're in the endoscopy suite, and just before she drifts off she says, I just know this will make it easier in life.

And at the same time I am sitting with the new knowledge that Dr. Talkington in 1999 did not dilate anything. Not a damn thing. And it throws us smack dab in the breach.

Where to go? I know what the academics would ask: What do you think you are doing? There is no clear indication for endoscopy and certainly no indication for dilation. Her X-ray showed no large collection of air in the stomach, and you haven't done a gastric emptying study yet.

The behavioralists would say, There is a belief system going here. Don't screw it up. She is deeply reliant upon you and your compassion for her condition, so much so that any act that is not harmful and contains within it an action of good intent is worth trying.

It's true. What have I ever done for this lady other than listen to her plight, show interest in rather than disgust at an unsolvable problem that threatens the ego of most doctors, search with her for some small alteration that will change the shape of her universe? Whatever that amounts to is the thread that makes it work. This is the source of her enthusiasm as she leaves my office, her courage as she takes long trips with her husband to Scandinavia, and the hope that allows her to keep going. Don't you retire, she says. I'll come to your house.

What will you find if you do? I almost say. Probably not what she expects. There's the game and then there are the players behind the game. Depends on what you want to know. And I remember, what was it? Ah yes, sham surgery, that was it, that nothing, that nonoperation they did to people who had abdominal pain. The surgeon opened the patient's belly and then didn't do a goddamn thing except let in a little stale operating room air and then close up again. And — surprise, surprise — almost without exception the patient got better. Go figure. Dramatic little trick, that was. Couldn't do it these days, but I'll be a monkey if it didn't work.

Okay. We are clear. I turn to her as she is falling to sleep. You're going to love this dilation, I say.

And I begin the endoscopy that I know will find nothing to dilate. Somehow, though, through the mere benevolence of invasion, the vitamin of action, something good will come from this, even if it is nothing more than the affirmation that says, *I am doing something for you.*

My scope whistles through the chambers, which open like curtains of modesty that know it is time to open, open to the knower and keeper of the secret, the architectures of normalcy that accompany chronic pain, these windless chambers inhabited by ghosts of worry, ghouls of sorrow and anxiety. My scope will aspirate the smoke of their habitation into my suction pot and discard it into the outer universe. I have become an alchemist under my cloak of modern medicine.

I will play my role. It is important I do so. I will tell her it was a great success.

And then I will wait for her phone call.

Blood Butterfly

only the truest things always
are true because they can't be true
— E. E. CUMMINGS

We were in bed when the call came in. Eight o'clock, Christmas morning.

She was dead when they found her, it said.

Oh my, I said, and I handed the phone to Joan.

She grumbled the way a person who is more asleep than awake grumbles when startled prematurely and before knowing, in this case, the reason would be so heavy. The phone was suspended a moment in air as if to question necessity, but it would not withdraw.

It was Amy on the line, Joan's sister. The "they" who found her were Joan's brother and his family, who were on a mission to visit a someone who was ill. That someone was their mother.

Our own children were asleep in their beds, the excitement of Christmas almost palpable under the swelling surface of their near waking, not yet ruptured into the day. I didn't know how the day might play out, but I did know we would conduct ourselves as closely as we could to the perfection we had planned before the message, holding its contents mute and sacred until its time.

Joan was off the phone.

She must have known she was dying, she said. She was in her bed with her will and all her papers.

There was a pause that wanted nothing more than the space it occupied.

Blood was everywhere, she whispered.

Some information you absorb without comment, as no comment is capable. Some you absorb as something distant, suddenly closer, slides deliberately in.

Joan would be of two minds now, a split fractal — one of maximum sorrow, the other of delight. I would see her at spots through the day spaced-out, the body arrested at its station, paralyzed and slack-jawed, while the mind spiraled in and out of the vortex of injury, a caesura of suspension between gifts, opened this time with a rough, chalky swirl of emotion.

If the children noticed anything, they didn't say as we piled articulately through the treasures of the most wonderful day of the year. A ten year old and a six year old — we weren't going to tell them, not yet.

Granny Jo had just visited us at Thanksgiving, her presence still hovering over the household like a long echo, her laughter at the Victor Borge video, her projects with the kids collecting plant specimens from the yard, her early morning cigarettes on the patio . . .

For two years now Joan knew, the way you just know things about the ones you love, that something was dreadfully wrong — a little edge of fatigue in her mother's voice, some reluctance to come and visit that was new and hard to define. Without the mathematics of truth it could still be felt niggling at us like a forgotten responsibility circling through the months in which she tried to get her mother to see a doctor, tried to get her to come west to visit our medical facility . . . *just get a checkup somewhere,* we had said to each other over and over again as we wrestled with intervention in the face of inexplicable resistance. But all the urgent entreaties had been deflected.

I know Joan thinks I have a death wish, Jo had said to me over Thanksgiving dishes at the kitchen sink, but I don't. I just accept what comes.

So the "what comes" had, by the time it was named, moved her from the square named diagnosis to the one named hospice all in one swift, unbroken move of the token. That's when she finally told her children, letting it slip in tidbits like gossip at a bridge party, indirect, discreet in the "oh, by the way" sort of tradition.

Okay if I see what I can do with my intelligent consultants? I had asked her.

Now that it's out in the open I don't see why not, she said. But we are really pretty far advanced here.

I know, I said, envisioning the mass expanding into the abdomen, reaching for distant organs . . .

It's at least a 3B or more by now, she said with the same tone of voice as if she were describing news reports of a political rally in Pakistan.

The presents opened themselves one by one. Neither the boys nor the process needed much from us as Joan and I endured the gush of memory and shock surging against our silence. Decisions formed themselves in the nonconversations we were having. Evolutions that take time were taking no time. Who would go? When would they go? Duston had his microscope, Gabriel his radio-control plane. We were taking a little pause for breakfast and, as is our custom, to stretch the pleasures as long as they will go. Joan was deciding what plane flight, what arrangement . . .

Washing my hands before breakfast was an act of vamping, waiting for Joan's emotions and plans to spill.

When one is encumbered by a daze, something usually rises up to take over. As I was drying my hands, Duston walked up. He said, Do you want to hear a legend?

This is about as unexpected and incongruent as him asking, Do you like raspberries on toast?

Sure, we said, having no idea whatsoever why we said it or what we were facing.

You know, people don't bleed to death, he said.

As I watched him saying this I tried to be sure I recognized what he said. I tried to be sure I recognized him. It *was* Duston, shifting his body around his words as he always does, speaking as if from the restless energy that somehow seems trapped and inexhaustible in his body.

But the message! I looked at Joan. The reaction that was incredulous at the message was large enough to be incredulous at the messenger.

He was still speaking, words moving on down the line of ideas even before we had time to catch up.

People don't bleed to death, he said. The Blood Butterfly comes and slowly takes their life away.

Our jaws dropped.

As a physician I am aware that there is a physiological aspect to our being we can predict and a mysterious, perhaps spiritual aspect we cannot. I see the mysterious in the way some people heal faster than others. I see it rise in us and bend us certain ways as we are confronted with illness or mortality, as if it waits for this, as if mystery always intends to rise up when we least expect it. Even so, Duston gave me two astonishments: how and at what level did he know? And how could he so quickly, perhaps even without knowing why, find a way to lift sorrow into beauty?

Our minds reviewed the events of the morning, remembering that we woke him from his sleep after the message came and concluded, as we must, there was no way he could know what had happened to Granny Jo — or the gory specifics we had heard but not spoken.

In the force field of Duston's legend, speech wanted not to be recovered. Yet I forced it open with a question. Where did that story come from? I asked.

I just made it up, he said.

And I don't know what we did in that moment. Perhaps we patted him on the back, and maybe we said a few words about how beautiful his legend was without giving it so much attention as to arouse worry, and then turned our attention to breakfast and the slippage of the day. Even so, the arrival of this moment, as had the one of the phone call, tunneled its way into our every gesture and urge.

All day Granny Jo's death stood apart, separate but not separate, untold and yet somehow astonishingly told, and still the specter in the room had not been introduced. It would stand there anonymously, with neither eyes nor voice, while neither of the boys would know until six days later, when Joan returned from Florida, a trip she ostensibly took because "Granny Jo was sick," parceling out sorrow from Christmas pleasures.

Christmas went. And had been marked without intending to be marked. Joan left on the red-eye Christmas night, and the boys and I entertained ourselves through the week, going to movies, playing tennis, experimenting with the new playthings, the boys still believing that Granny Jo was sick somewhere and her children were gathering to take care of her.

I guess they were doing just that.

Then one day Joan returned with her sorrow and her news. Duston cried for an hour. All that time he had lived with his suspension and his newly forged legend, not knowing the connection between the two or suspecting the pathway that made them part of each other, protective of each other, that very separation lifting him somehow through his question, how's Granny Jo, how's Granny Jo . . . his other self, the one who already knew and had spoken its knowledge, waiting for him to name it and pull it in.

Is Something Wrong with Your Prostate?

Does he have something wrong with his prostate? And is he doing something about it?

Now I know what you're thinking. I'd think the same thing if I read a sentence like that. You'd say to yourself, Well, that might be lifted from a conversation between two doctors or between a doctor and the wife of one of his patients. Something like that. Or maybe it's someone expressing concern about someone else not showing enough concern. Maybe that.

Not that at all. It's my patient talking about *me*.

Give her the gold star for the day, that's what I said. I've never heard anything like *that* before. *Do I have something wrong with my prostate*. I love that!

So now let's back up a bit and see if I can explain any of this.

Okay. So she comes to see me last week. This was after she called a few times requesting lab tests she wanted to have run. *Few*, I say. She wanted her liver tested, and her spleen (I'm not sure how to do that), and then she wanted to know if her minerals were in balance and if that balance filtered down to her colon, and then there was a request for a test to see if her digestive enzymes were all okay.

Whoa, I said. What am I, a short-order cook?

So I made her come to the office. We need to make some sense of this, I said.

So she's already mad. To think that she has to discuss when she already *knows* what she wants.

The visit was nice enough. I wanted to know what symptoms she had.

Well, she just wanted to make sure everything was all right.

But what makes you think it isn't?

Well, I read somewhere that your system can be out of balance.

What makes you think yours is?

Things are not working right.

What's not working right?

I don't know.

Then why do you think some tests will be abnormal?

I don't.

Then why do you want to get them?

Well, they might be.

She was smiling. I was smiling. And we were getting absolutely nowhere. A doctor has to have something to work with besides the *notion* that something might be wrong.

Symptoms, I said.

What about them?

Do you have any?

I don't know.

Well, what do you feel?

That things are not right.

The thought occurred to me that we had been here before, right here in this very same spot, as a matter of fact, and instead of following the deductive, articulate course that most productive conversations in a doctor's office are supposed to take and, I assume, *try* to take and that might, with a little bit of luck, push things in the direction of a solution, we were spinning around like a top, going nowhere and apparently incapable of correcting ourselves.

Well, can't I just have a CBC?

And I'm thinking that everyone, even people who cannot come up with any good symptoms whatsoever, might deserve to have a complete blood count now and then.

Oh well, sure, I said.

And chemistries? How about chemistries?

Any particular ones you have in mind?

And now it finally occurs to me that I am not in charge here. Not in the slightest. I am an academic, for Christ's sake, trained in the very best manner in the very best institutions. Apparently, all that good reasoning doesn't protect me from paralysis at the hands of the self-convinced illogical. I am not in charge. Not that *she* is. Apparently, *nobody* is.

Well, we made a little list of things to do like the Thursday shopping list at the 7-Eleven and I agreed to most everything because it seemed not unreasonable even if I didn't know the reason, and then I felt a little sheepish, feeling like something had happened here that all my good planning wasn't fully in touch with, so I thought that the best thing to do was for all of us to get up and leave the room real quick before any more tests showed up on this list of ours.

So I did that.

And she followed. And how about lead poisoning? she said.

Do you think you have been poisoned?

Well, things . . .

. . . are not right, I know, I know.

And I actually agreed to a heavy metal screen in spite of good solid academic training that should have taught me better. I think my brain must have been dead doornail numb. There was a manner of thinking at work here that was tracking off in another direction, an unfamiliar direction in which the rules were unapparent or perhaps known only to the tracker. How can you talk to the guide if you don't speak the language?

And how about . . .

. . . wait a minute.

No, really. I'd like to know about my enzymes.

What enzymes?

My digestive enzymes.

What about them?

Are they working as they should be.

You look healthy to me. You're not losing weight.

But they seem not to be working right.

Well, I sure as hell wasn't going to chase after that. I doubt it, I said. Anyway, the only way to test enzymes like that — other than through some indirect evidence we garner from general nutritional tests, which we have, no doubt, more than adequately covered — is to drop a tube down into your stomach and drag out some goo and then run a few tests on it in somebody's Goo Lab, and then we can see if the enzymes are doing their job.

I thought that little description might slow down the conversation a bit.

It did have that effect.

But then she looked at me like I didn't know what the hell I was talking about.

Funny thing is, she was partly right. Having failed the rational defenses, I might have stooped to a bit of the irrational myself.

I don't think you'd want that, I said, trying to recover some of the impact I'd hoped to accomplish.

Aren't there any other tests we should run?

No.

No?

I think we've got it covered.

That was *not* good news. The object, just in case I missed it, was not to finish the list, because the list was at its very best when opening directly out into the universe.

But I've read somewhere . . .

In that moment I almost challenged her to declare whether she was more inclined to believe me and the "science" I was trying to represent or to believe whoever this "I've read somewhere" person was, but I was pretty sure I already knew the answer to that.

So I found something I had to do right now, right immediately over in the other room, and I made a right hasty exit.

She hung around the office for another hour and a half, catching me between patients with this "I know what I want and you are *not* giving it to me" kind of look that I could neither dispel nor avoid, but I stood my ground.

Now she calls to complain to my receptionist that I was not cooperative and that I was a very poor doctor and did I have something wrong with my prostate.

And then, boys and girls, she left her telephone number.

Christ!

Well, you know I just *had* to call her up.

Hi, this is Dr. Watts.

Oh, thank you for calling. So the questions I have left for you: First of all, I'll come right out . . . were you joking around? I thought you were joking around, tubes out the bottom and stuff . . .

No, no, not out the bottom. You mean to measure the enzymes you were talking about?

Yes.

No, not out the bottom, for heaven's sake, the mouth, the mouth.

Oh, so you meant out the mouth. So we weren't joking.

No, not if you want to measure the enzymes directly.

And the neutrophil count was the opposite way?

Opposite way?

You said when I said it was off one point that it was the opposite way?

I felt like I was trying to explain the game of cricket to a West Texas cowboy. What I said was — so here I go — that if the white count were up, that would be an indication of infection or inflammation. If it were down, usually that is still okay, unless it is really low, in which case you might be susceptible to infection.

Well, I don't want to go into that now ... How did the lab come out?

The lab tests were all just fine.

All okay, well, that's good. Even though they were normal, the WBC I mean, I wanted to see if *E. coli* was there.

They're always there if you're talking about the colon.

Yeah but, oh well, never mind. Regarding the ... I thought you were really laughing.

Laughing?

Laughing about the tubes.

No.

When I asked the lab they said it was a blood test.

That's to measure the enzymes *in*directly. You can measure the blood levels of protein, glucose, fat, stuff like that — but to measure them directly ...

So why do they bother doing that test? Anyway, I'll let that go, because you are the expert and maybe I'm the native fool. Anyway, when I left the office I was so confused I decided to cancel my colonoscopy.

I had forgotten we'd scheduled a colonoscopy, but I wasn't going to argue.

I wanted to ask you if you were all right because I was really confused when I was in your office and we were talking about where it got released to the neutrophil and you said it was the intestine ...

Oh, I remember. You're talking about the circulation of blood going from the gastrointestinal tract to the liver rather than the vena cava.

Oh, so it didn't have anything to do with the neutrophil?

Not that I know of.

Conversation tracks were overlapping. There was a melting of information across subject matters, and it was unclear at times which track we were on. I thought I had better do my little inquiry, which seems to have been motivated by an unquenchable curiosity, before I got further distracted. Why was I in this conversation this long? Anyway...

You asked something about a prostate?

Oh, prostate, yes. Oh, I'm real embarrassed. I said that because when I left your office I was so confused I said he must be laughing. Laughing. You know, sometimes when men ... well, you know, the men they have prostate problems like women have menopause and sometimes men have, well, you know, prostate mental problems...

Prostate mental problems?

Yes, well, I was worried.

That's funny, I said. What are prostate mental problems?

Well, I didn't know. I just wondered if you should get checked out or something, but maybe, I don't know, maybe this woman is coming from a higher state of consciousness or is very confused or something, I ... Anyway, I'll do the colonoscopy sometime later and thank you very much, good-bye.

So that was it. She wasn't off base in her assessment; I was. And since logic can follow after any false assumption, she was diagnosing my prostate by way of my brain, the culprit responsible for the glitch in the orderly procession toward her beloved enzyme tests. Neat trick to see the physiology of that miserable little organ through the aura of my mental behavior and give it all the blame.

Learn a little somethin' every day. Prostate mental problems, yes indeedy.

Was it worth it to have pursued it this far? Didn't I know this way of thinking would land bizarre? Yes, I did, but which bizarre, that's the deal.

Well, I know you thought it was finished. But it's not.

My administrator walks into the room just now, and she says that she was just on the phone with "that woman" again. It was just too much, she said. And then she made some spinning-around-the-head motions with both hands.

What did she want?

I don't know. That's why I asked her to write you a letter. I couldn't follow her, something about tubes coming out of her head...?

The Soft Animal of the Body

You just have to let the soft animal of the body
Love what it loves.
— MARY OLIVER

Arriving at the endo suite for my own colonoscopy, I was relaxed and comfortable. I do these every day myself. I know the limits. I know the safeties. On top of that, I've had one before. It's a known thing.

In my mind the voice of confidence was speaking, saying that very soon will come the vital feeling of accomplishment that follows a difficult but purposeful task, as if a small diploma signifying emotional vigor had been given, one that assures protection from colon cancer for another five to ten years. Now that I have done what I should to avoid the doctor's trap — ignoring the self while caring for others — my small children will be very happy. And I will be happy for their sake.

Blood pressure 140/86, I heard the nurse say.

Zooks! That's thirty points high. I guess I'm more pumped than I thought.

The nurse just raised her eyebrows.

I zoned back into my relaxation mode, my life-is-great mode, my I'm-so-glad-to-be-here mode.

My doctor, my colleague, my choice, was filling out the papers. These days that process takes almost as long as the procedure itself. It interested me how he dealt with the awkward time that writing all that stuff manufactures. His method was silence. I measured my own way of joking and teasing against his.

Now the gurney ride. I have wondered how this felt, ceiling going by, walls partly visible, traveling by way of the safe arms of those who tend me. Some chariot, I say. I know, I know, humor — a way of dealing.

Then the beginning. I have chosen no anesthetic, no sedation. It should be noted that if a patient of mine asks for no sedation, he is usually a doctor. Or sometimes a pilot or an accountant. These occupations have in common being control freaks.

Foolish, this no sedation business, the nurses think. It gets me another eyebrow raise. Affectionate condemnation, I am sure. But then I have patients waiting across the street. Ha *ha!*

Now the expected cramping of the scope and air, the somewhat unexpected plunge and withdrawal feeling at the mouth to the outer world — but I have been here before, I say to myself, yet the body does not remember. Or maybe it does, better so than I do.

We are now passing the little spasms of the descending colon, roadblocks the body throws up as if to say, Wait a goddamn minute, here. A little water, my doctor says, makes the cramp go away. I feel a cinch at the spot where my grandfather might have located the gizzard, and I laugh under my now-somewhat-strictured breath. We are moving forward, yes indeed!

About here is where I turn the patient on his back, a maneuver to lessen the drag of gravity across the transverse colon and thus minimize the pressure against the walls of the bowel. Easier for both the endoscopist and the patient.

I suggest it.

It's okay, my doctor says. Which means no thank you and which hits me like, well, okay for *him,* maybe.

The nurse was looking at the monitor. Heart rate 129, she said softly and, at the same time, menacingly.

My doctor nodded.

He started at 67, she added.

Nothing more was said.

I had the growing sensation that I wanted to be somewhere else, to have this over with.

I began to review the last conversation. Or lack thereof. Yes, we could finish despite the wide changes in heart rate, but what about the cardiovascular system in the meanwhile? Just like a doctor to be tuned in to both sides of the conversation and have them try their best to scare each other.

He was taking his time. Doing a good job. Maybe he's right, I thought. I'll defer to his style. He's done almost as many of these as I have.

The nurse had become animated. I was concentrating on other things. Pulse rate 40, she said, and highly irregular. The EKG machine stuck out a tongue of paper all the way to the floor. My doctor seemed not to notice.

How do you feel? asked the nurse.

I wasn't sure. And I couldn't tell how much the question was asked to really want to know the answer and how much it was asked to alert the doctor, who hadn't paid any attention so far, to the subtleties of an erratic heart rate.

A little strange perhaps, I answered. My toughness struggled with my chickenness over the words to choose. I decided to let the answer decide for itself. It wanted to continue: A little light-headed, I added, perhaps.

The nurse lowered my head, a trained response to the early stages of shock.

Time to stop, I said, as if from nowhere in particular. The words just popped out and surprised especially me. If I had had time or inclination I would have tried to imagine where that voice had come from.

No response.

George, I said.

Yeah.

And while I was figuring out what to say, the voice took over: PULL IT OUT.

There was a delay, then a soft, Yeah.

The nurse asked if I felt any better.

I couldn't say that I did, for whatever had been disturbed stayed disturbed, so I could only commit to an unconvincing maybe.

George was still fiddling around in the ascending colon.

My body took over and rolled itself halfway on its back, stretching out a bit. I was beyond courtesy. My body cared nothing for courtesy.

And he did start pulling out, though very slowly, I thought.

I was putty.

Some time passed. I may even have pulled on the scope myself.

I'm going to send you to the recovery room, the nurse said when he finally finished. I think you'd better stay with us awhile.

I lay very still and concentrated on the task: to gather myself back into myself. It felt like part of me had oozed out and puddled in the bed beside me.

Your color is better.

Thirty minutes had passed. It was the recovery nurse speaking.

You were white as a sheet when you came in here. Do you feel like getting up?

Sure, I said. And in the same instant lay right back down. Not even the slightest upward tilt of the bed was imaginable.

Flat, I said.

And they did that.

Well, at least your oxygen saturation stayed okay, she said.

I was thinking how in this situation, that of the first sustained low heart rate, I would have been out of that colon in a flash. A different appreciation of risk? A difference of style, I told myself.

Then I wondered: could it be that my style is determined by

what the soft animal of my body knows about itself, knows about what it can take and cannot? And what it fears? I was astonished to learn that, despite my comfort with the whole idea of colonoscopy, my body had a very different take on the process. Not only that, it behaved in a manner independent from my thinking. The idea began to appear to me that sedation, even for control freaks, maybe especially for control freaks, is a good thing.

Men! the recovery nurse was saying, her words and her laughter breaking the thin shell of my cocoon. You think you can do this.

Whereupon she turned on her heel and left me to my juices.

Let the body love what it loves, says Mary Oliver. What about fear what it fears?

My psychiatrist friends tell me that the evolution of fear is well founded: our inherited aversion to spiders, snakes, confined spaces, and precipices have rolled themselves into our genes as ingrained, automatic responses that are connected to matters of survival. It's when, as they say, we use our rational brain to talk ourselves out of fear, climbing into a stranger's car, for example, that bad things happen.

No doubt that's so. But what about the things we have to do anyway, things that are frightening but necessary, good for us even though we cannot love doing them?

My neocortex has no doubts. My soft animal does.

Meanwhile, the nurse has left. She knows that in time my body will right itself, will reattach itself to the mind, which it has rejected in a fit of pique and which now has other thoughts. Later, and together, they will stand up and walk out as if nothing happened.

In the meantime my heart rate goes up and then down like some wild flailing of incensed protest, my head feels light, and I am trying to speak to the little animal who will take no words of assurance.

She needs more time. And all the while she is sending messages of anger, of agitation, a not-so-playful *yaka-yaka-yaka*, scolding her intruders. Hardwired, as she is, to my autonomic nervous system, she is scrambling electrical impulses, which crackle around inside me like the Morse code of distress. I will wait it out and plan to reward the little creature first chance I get . . .

Maybe a cold glass of Chardonnay . . .

Maybe a promise or two . . .

Aspirin and Beauty

I'm a castoff from the cardiologist, said the lanky white-haired research scientist. Then he gave his cowboy hat a little flick with his forefinger, an affectation I thought surprisingly fitting despite his distinctly Slavic accent. He gave me a mournful look.

Seen it before, I said.

Well, he did every test known to mankind and then some. Then he said nothing was wrong with my heart.

Good news, I said.

Yeah, but the problem's still there.

So let's start over. What problem?

Chest pain.

Figures.

How so?

Chest pain. Well, people think first of the heart. It's natural. The most scary thing comes to mind first. But most chest pain has nothing to do with the heart. Still, people go to cardiologists first, so, naturally, there is a steady stream from those guys to the gastroenterologist.

Why is that?

Well, did you think of your esophagus when you got your chest pain?

I see your point.

Few people do. And it's hard to tell the two, heart pain and esophagus pain, apart. Even those who have both diseases can't tell the difference sometimes.

That's not fair.

Same nerves transmit the message of pain from the esophagus and from the heart. The two pains can mimic each other exactly, even to the point of radiating up to the chin or out over the left arm.

Heart's okay.

So now to the esophagus. What does the pain feel like?

Sharp.

Not burning?

Not.

Does it happen at night or after eating?

Mostly when I change position.

That's not sounding like heart *or* esophagus. Where is it exactly?

Right here over my heart.

Use one finger.

Gee, that's hard.

Do it anyway. It's important.

Okay.

And he struggled to find the place to land his finger but waffled awhile before eventually resting it over the fourth rib just as it makes its curve toward the sternum.

Just there?

Just there.

Now, what position makes it worse?

Twisting, mostly. Like when I turn to look behind me in the car.

Sounds musculoskeletal.

What does that mean?

Coming from the support structures of the body. Let's walk this through.

Okay.

Heart pain — angina — feels like an elephant standing on your chest. It stops you in your tracks, radiates to the shoulder and arm, and can be associated with sweating, shortness of breath, and, as they say in textbooks, a fear of impending doom.

That's not me.

Esophagus can go into spasm if it gets roughed up enough by stomach acid. And that little squeeze can imitate heart pain almost to the letter.

I don't have indigestion.

Definitely against esophagus. But people are wired differently, and some don't feel indigestion until the esophagus gets so irritated that it goes nutcracker.

Not me.

Probably. So we might be able to do without an endoscopy here after all.

Oh goody.

I thought you'd like that. But we're not done yet. Listen to this: a judge from Modesto came to see me for hoarseness. Turns out he had esophagitis to his earlobes and never had one solitary symptom.

Except hoarseness.

Right.

I prefer that "not esophagus" stuff. Let's stick to that. But if it's not esophagus, what is it then?

I looked at him and tried to decide if I should go playful or serious. Given that choice I'll always pick playful. Tsetse syndrome, I said.

You mean the fly.

Same name, different thing.

You've lost me.

Take off your shirt and I'll show you.

He did.

Now lie down.

I hope you know what you're doing.

You'd be surprised.

I can't wait.

Okay, let's see if we can reproduce the pain.

I place my finger on the spot he pointed to and push gently.

Ow.

That was easy.

Easy for you.

Costochondritis.

What's that?

Tsetse syndrome.

Doc-*tor!*

Okay, okay. There's a little joint here between the end of the rib and the piece of cartilage that connects it to the breastbone. That's what allows you to move your rib cage — that basket of bones — when you breathe. There's an inflammation that sets up in here sometimes, right at that joint. That process makes for pain, which you, because you think that anything in your chest overlying your heart has to do with some mortal disease, immediately think heart attack.

That's what I did.

Everybody does that, even doctors who should know better. When chest pain hits the brain, we immediately imagine the worst.

Why do I have that?

Some virus you may not even have recognized landed there after it had done whatever it was programmed to do elsewhere in your body. Or maybe somebody hugged you too hard . . .

Unlikely.

. . . and snapped a little crack in the junction right here.

Just had to be over my heart, didn't it?

Just had to be. Besides, you've probably perpetuated it.

How so?

Well, think about it. What's the first thing you're going to do when you have chest pain and you think you have a heart condition?

How about worry like hell?

Exactly. And that turns up the volume.

I see.

And doesn't allow it to slide away into nothingness as it should.

I don't see.

Pain begets pain.

Mmmmm.

Okay. I'll tell you a story. A man had pancreatitis with severe pain. For a lot of reasons they had to take his pancreas out. After the operation he still had the pain.

Maybe they missed the diagnosis.

Try this: a man had his leg shot off in Vietnam. He still has pain in the big toe that he doesn't have anymore.

Phantom pain.

Pain can develop a life of its own, rise up the spinal column, and spin around in those vaporous chambers of the brain even after the affected part is no longer around.

You're scaring me.

No. Yours is gonna go away.

Why?

First, because we gave it a name. If I had called it John the Baptist it would get better just because we called it something.

Wasn't he beheaded?

Listen. The poets of Ireland used to be called bards. They got their power over stuff by their ability to name things. They drove out devils, deinfested houses overrun with rats and stuff.

Now he was looking at me wide-eyed.

Don't discount it. There is power in the ability to put a name on something.

This is sounding like the Twilight Zone.

No, it's probably internal. We feel better, the subconscious feels better, if whatever's bothering us has a name.

He nodded.

Second, this pain is no longer connected to the fear of sudden death from a heart attack, which takes down its power source. Without that, it's going to fizzle and die.

How long? he asked.

How long has it been there?

Well, actually about a month.

Rib cage takes a long time. Did you have a viral infection to start out?

No.

Some don't.

Well, I did have a cold a couple of weeks before.

See there. That could have done it.

Really, a cold?

Yeah. Some little something to set it off, and then you're checking in on it all the time, giving it attention because you're afraid of the heart thing, and that attention plus the fact that you press on it from time to time causes it to grow or stay longer than it should, and the first thing you know, the mind-body connection is working in the wrong direction. All we need to do is to switch the electrical charge, and we're halfway there.

You make it sound simple.

Oh it is, mostly. Occasionally, we have to do a little drama.

Drama?

In the service I had a staff sergeant who, a long time before, had a collapsed lung. It gave him chest pain right about the spot where yours is. The pneumothorax went away. Gone bye-bye. Only problem, he kept getting the pain and thinking the lung had collapsed all over again. Like flashbacks. Like the body got this cantankerous signal stuck in its memory. But it hadn't come back. So we shot a little Novocain in there to break the cycle, and he was good and quiet for a while. Truth is, I don't know if the Novocain or the drama with needle and drug was what made it all better, but it don't much matter. It worked.

I think I'll avoid that little deal.

If you find yourself in that condition, you'll be asking for that little deal. But like I say, you're going to get better.

And as I said that I realized part of what I was doing was adding another drug to the mix: the drug called Expectation. The reassurance and positive outlook that go with it were better than a flu shot. It reminded me of the dean of students I sent to the cardiologist for hypertension management. The cardiologist put one hand on his shoulder and said, We're going to do just fine here. Of all the things the cardiologist had said and done, only that impressed the dean enough for him to tell me about it.

Are you practicing medicine or witchcraft?

Both.

Aren't you going to be run out of the AMA?

Not these days. Besides, both are what's required. And make no mistake. If there's a mechanical or biologic problem here, we'll have to fix it before things will get better. But in this case I think the body will work its own magic.

I'm sitting here thinking that I'm not into pain. So why do I have this?

You have good reason for it. There's injury or inflammation there. But if it keeps going, there may be some multipliers attached. If that's the case, we'll deal with it later. For now let's assume it's going away.

Assumption made.

Meanwhile, a little heat, a little anti-inflammatory meds if you need them, and then concentrate on something beautiful.

Take two aspirin and call me in the morning?

Something beautiful and call me in the morning.

I knew that's all I'd get from you.

You want surgery?

No thanks.

Endoscopy?

He saluted. Not this buckaroo.

Sometimes the job of the doctor is to stand in the way of things to be done.

Like all that cardiology stuff?

Maybe. But look, this little discussion has stopped endoscopy, CT scan of the chest — you know, dollars and probes.

Okay. I'm with you. Aspirin and something beautiful?

Aspirin and beautiful.

Think that'll do it, Doc?

It's worked for centuries.

Notes from the Center of
a Perpetual Breakdown

*Everybody has their story. Even in the
most improbable of circumstances they
want their story told.* — JOHN BURNS,
New York Times bureau chief, Iraq

God gave you to me. That's what he said.

She had come in and out of my practice. She had come in and
out of my office. She actually worked in my office for a time, fil-
ing, sorting, a something-just-to-keep-her-occupied kind of project that she would refer to years later as being my "office manager
without pay."

She had some indeterminate kind of illness that made her
matchstick thin and constipated to the hilt. About the time she
was dying the first time she entered my life. Her mother did too,
though I never met her. Or at least I don't think I ever did, even
though Chacon kept telling me she was gorgeous and wondered
openly if any man including me could resist her.

This relationship she had with her mother was by all accounts
mutually destructive — the telephone calls that inquired intru-
sively about her bowel habits, the accusations of poor self-care,
the justifications that rang hollow in the icy deep freeze of the
mother's countenance ("Don't thank me, it's just something else I
will do to help my own daughter"). These offerings did not steady
the hemorrhaging or soothe the wound that connected the two of
them but instead kept it pulled open in the stinging air.

I was an escort, she said. I don't know if you ever knew that
about me. I was intelligent and good-looking and I was conver-

sational. Men loved to take me places and paid well to do that. I dressed well. I was discreet. All this was going on when I first met you, but I don't think you knew about it. I just knew from your voice I needed to stay where you were.

My wife at the time fired her. Actually, I did, but I blamed it, conveniently, on the person *not* present in my office. Chacon was sparring with my secretary and a few other people around the office, and since it was an arrangement of convenience designed for her, and since the balance of good things and not-so-good things had gone south, the whole thing just needed to go away.

Thirty years later she weighs 78 pounds, lives in an apartment that sweats water from the ceiling and floor, at least according to the thirty-minute messages my office answering tape records some five or six times a day, times like 11:30 P.M., 11:59 P.M., 3:50 A.M., 4:45 A.M. . . .

Friday, February 18, 5:57 P.M. This is for Juan, Dr. Watts's secretary. Thank you for your call this morning. When you called, water, Juan, you know, water W-A-T-E-R from the rainstorm is coming through my ceiling and into other apartments next door to me — right over the telephone. I couldn't hold to get a pen. I would have been electrocuted. The phone blew up. This is a different telephone. It short-circuited. I . . . couldn't use the phone all day, so, and there's still water coming through my ceiling. Would you make a note of that for my medical records, for David, because my landlord does not give us a safe place to live. I will try. If you are open Monday you can call me to give me the schedule. Thank you for calling, really it was a terrible emergency, there's still water coming through my ceiling. I'm sorry I couldn't talk, but one minute later the phone went, like, on fire. Okay, thank you. Bye-bye.

I have sent social workers to her apartment, but she kicks them out. I sent a visiting nurse, who, Chacon says, is incompetent. Chacon wants me to talk to the mayor because he has a program that might find her housing on the basis of "profound need." But she has refused any housing we have found for her, and I am not in the business of finding housing in the first place. I have no qualifications for finding housing. I tell her this and she says, Well, if you'd just fill out this one more form . . .

Wednesday, January 26, 6:43 P.M. There was this one person with her lack of English, and then, at the end, Charles. Chris was very quiet. But we all agreed that Sarah and I were not a good mesh. She didn't listen to a thing they said and while holding the power of medical attorney that Dr. Applebarth said could cancel my sister's power of attorney. She did not want to look at any of the doctor's reports. You could pretty much read her. She had on designer clothing and she said she had never spoken to me before and when I showed her the notes of the times she called she was very embarrassed. She left me with everything that I've already done, housing lists for independent housing. There's an agent and I have to prove, and as you know we don't know if I'm on any lists, David, I have a question I would like to ask you. I am planning to pay one month's rent. I have an appointment for the one test . . . Could you give me a doctor the surgeon a call I can hardly speak and talk tomorrow because my diagnosis . . . is not good. END OF MESSAGE. TO REPEAT THIS MESSAGE PRESS 1. TO SAVE IT PRESS 2. TO ERASE . . .

———

Wednesday, January 26, 8:45 P.M. David, I'm just going take a risk and finish this message time is anyhow without a secretary today but I didn't need a secretary I go for a long period of time without speaking . . .

. . . I went to work under the child Mann, M-A-N-N, Act which was later abolished because it gave such high benefits except for vision and dental which I can't even seek if I need Neurontin which aren't covered at my age and he said that my reasons for request could be a reasonable one, and it seems the only way I'm going to get that, David, just to let you put me in Laguna Honda Hospital which everyone said was not very nice and, uh, again I was very moved by him and the aftercare . . .

... I have an ET so I've pretty much made my decision but there was a medical student in the room so I did not tell you I write, when you say I should write, I write, David, I write at least six to twelve hours a day it's how I survived, despite my horrible handwriting, I also memorized the manuscript, I memorized the manuscript so my sister couldn't take that from me. Now that I know the passport I would like maybe perhaps to take the money from the third month's rent and go to Israel and rest there. I'd like to speak with you about that. I'm very tired ... END OF MESSAGE. TO REPEAT THIS MESSAGE PRESS 1. TO SAVE IT ...

So I tell my secretary I'm puzzled whether Chacon really wants my help or she just wants to be in my life. On the surface of it, it seems to be a desperate situation, and she seems to be dedicated to the prospect of solving it, and yet the solutions that arrive are rejected out of hand.

And I remember Chacon saying more than once, If someone would just give me a place in the basement, just one room with a bathroom, I could take care of their kids and not interfere in the private life of the family ... just a tent in the backyard would be better than where I am living now. Do you know anyone like that? I'm not suggesting that *you* should do this, of course.

Well, of course she was. And if I would let her, she would insinuate herself into my house, my family, my breakfast table ... and I was absolutely certain that, like the ban I put on these so-long-I-can't-listen-to-all-of-them telephone calls, she would be out of control and in my face. In my children. It was unimaginable.

No, Chacon. I don't know anyone like that.

I limited her to twenty minutes a day of telephone space on my message tape. Whereupon she occupied two hours.

Thursday, January 27, 8:58 P.M. This message is for David Watts. David, I just finished speaking with Dr. Applebarth who called me tonight. At 7:30 this morning I called Charles Windom that came with the put-together-very-quickly-yesterday-morning group, unfortunately, as I mentioned to you, they sent this person who barely speaks English and while holding the copy of the power of attorney that Dr. Applebarth after my sister forged my signature derailing me from Berkeley Housing. You know you can get rid of sister's power of attorney? I was also told by her that I have to force my landlord and if it hadn't worked twenty-one twelve to identify what housing program it was there was of course it does not work by letters by Dr. Applebarth — you are a writer, David, you write magnificent letters. Dr. Applebarth is just doing what he can — when I spoke with him last Thursday he said he had no idea . . .

. . . Meanwhile, I, David, have what is termed Stockholm Syndrome and the whistling one in that. But we'll leave it at that as this is the message. And also posttronomic stress syndrome. In November of this year, in fact this is still going on, and I have volumes, volumes, David. But I did announce to Dr. Hatma the surgeon to please call you because I need the surgery but we're already got one test the CAT scan but I can't stand another . . . END OF MESSAGE. TO REPEAT THIS MESSAGE . . .

To ignore her pained my conscience. To pay attention anguished my professional standards. I wasn't clear that she needed surgery or wanted it. She was not anxious to have tests, but she was anxious to have surgery? It didn't make sense. She just seemed to want to get into the hospital. My secretaries were ready for the loony bin.

She might be just using the illusion of help to engage us, I said.

They were incredulous.

Look what happens if we deliver what she asks.

She refuses, they said, simultaneously.

Exactly. So . . . ?

Chacon started bringing in artifacts from her life. You should have these, she said.

I didn't understand why.

Here is the art portfolio of my father. He was a famous man, you know, the leading rabbi in Russia before immigrating to the

U.S. He became an artist and a philosopher. People came from miles around to hear his pronouncements. He was written up in the papers in New York. Don't you see what's there in his art? It's me, I'm the naked woman in the corner bleeding from the vagina, and here again as the snake with a woman's head. He never told me, but I know it.

How do you know it's you? I asked.

From his footsteps in the hall. And here's a picture of my sister at the bat mitzvah of her daughter. It was the last time I was there. She excommunicated me. Took over the inheritance. That's why I'm dirt poor and have nothing. I will run out of rent money in two months, David, if you don't do something to help me, I'll be out on the street.

I'm a doctor, I said. I will try, but I've sent people to you who are expert in these matters, and you keep getting rid of them. How come?

They're idiots. Can't you see what's going on, David? It's not difficult. I'm starving, I'm sick with polyhydromonial neurolical asthenia syndrome, with myositis, osteogenisis imperfecta . . . I went on the Internet with my diagnoses. I shouldn't even be alive by now.

Out my window the sun rises and the sun sets. The wind comes and sometimes rain. We limp along, even though she is pushing awfully hard against the accelerator, hard against the lever for attention and the lever for . . . what?

Listen to the first five minutes of each message, I tell my staff. If there is something new or dramatic or dangerous, listen to the rest, otherwise . . .

So they came to me saying she was threatening suicide.

What did she say?

We saved it for you. She says she wants to have permission to die.

How did she ask?

She wants a document that says . . .

I picked up the phone and called in the Emergency Life Crisis Intervention team. They already knew her name.

Chacon was furious.

I did not say suicide, she said. My primary doctor understands me much better than you do on this matter. He knows I would never kill myself. I am not religious, God forbid, but I would never do that. I'm surprised at you.

So I called the primary. He was a laid-back Texas hippie who was not sympathetic to my situation. Apparently, he was not besieged by Chacon the same way I was. I began finally to see all this as a matter of her *personal* attachment to me. Made it all the more dangerous. And now this neat little trap: I couldn't risk distance for fear of setting off her suicide/self-loathing tendencies, yet I had to guard against raging turmoil in my practice.

Dump her, my wife said.

She would be right. Two different wives, two *very different* wives, come to think of it, yet one and the same opinion.

I'm trying, I said.

Not hard enough, she said.

I had the feeling everything was up in the stratosphere, helium filled, about to rupture. None of this starting-out-on-the-ground business. We had started in rarefied air and then gotten higher. Day by day the same. So much calamity. She is starving, she is poor, she is dying . . .

She's been dying for twenty-five years, and she's not dead yet, my wife said. What do you make of that?

Right. I should pay attention to that. But then there's this suicide thing.

Just a threat.

Probably. Maybe I can set her down easy.

You dreamer.

The calls kept coming in. Implicit suicide remained in the picture, though it seemed that if we didn't talk about it, it wasn't really there, and meanwhile the artifacts accumulated like sticky rice in a wok.

My Crohn's is killing me, she said. I have pain. I can't eat. I get nauseous just thinking about food. I don't want to look like a broom straw, but between not being able to eat and not having enough money to buy food how can I catch up? I just eat a yogurt and a little bean curd and that's about it.

And I was thinking that's precisely what I don't know. And had not been able to find out all this time. Here I've learned more about her social disease than her medical one(s).

I'd like to do a few tests, I said.

Absolutely.

You see, I can't know what to do if I don't know the state of your disease.

Absolutely.

Medicine is a matter of balance, I was thinking. How much organic to the disease process and how much overlay from all the other stuff that makes us so interesting as humans — that distinction is what has to be sorted out. With Chacon it could be anything, and the frustrating part is, I could tell nothing on the basis of her symptoms. Besides being irrational, the symptoms wouldn't stand still. They shape-shifted, morphed, turned inside out, and, what's more, in spite of her dire circumstance they never were the center of conversation. If I forced them front and center, she resisted. If I brought them up, she demurred. When she mentioned them, she glided on past as if to protect them from scrutiny. Even though the reporting of symptoms is often like exploring the dark, in the case of Chacon it was more like picking up quicksilver.

I have in mind a small bowel follow-through and a colonoscopy, I said.

I don't know about that.

Of all the tests I could have chosen for you to have these are the simplest and will give us the most information.

They won't find my malabsorption.

If you have it, and if it is due to anything anatomical, it will.

David, I can't absorb food.

You have to absorb something, otherwise you'd be gone by now.

Nothing comes into my body.

I know these tests can be humiliating, but the small bowel follow-through is just swallowing barium and having the radiology folk follow it through. As for the colonoscopy, actually, it will be easier on you than on most people because of the colon surgery Dr. Constantino did for your constipation.

That surgery had occurred during the earlier iteration of *The David and Chacon Show*. The extreme and forced use of laxatives and enemas her mother threw at her had had damaging effects on her colon. It became sluggish. Consumed by torpor. It lay dead in the water. No laxative or combination thereof could dislodge the brickbats that clogged her system. So the operation that surgeons hate most because there is no "disease" to be taken out was done. Three-quarters of her colon was removed and hooked up again, small bowel to sigmoid. Then she had stools.

Because of all that your colonoscopy will take only five minutes, but it will offer us critical information about the general health of your gastrointestinal tract. Then I can know whether to treat your Crohn's disease or to look for some other reason for your problem.

And so the little dance began.

Schedule. Postpone. Schedule and postpone. Schedule and cancel. Or not show up. Swing to the left, then swing to the right. *Allemande left with your left hand, back to your partner with a right and left Grand.* Music could be written to this. Texas hoedown. Then a new twist: "Nobody told me so."

Chacon, we're getting nowhere.

I'm too sick.

That's precisely why we need to know.

I'm too busy trying to get my landlord to clean up the fungus in my apartment. Will you write him a letter?

I've already talked to him on the phone, and, in fact, he seems to be trying to do the best he can. He told me I was not the first doctor who called.

I can't afford it.

We've dealt with that already. I'm doing it practically for free. Whatever your MediCal and Medicare covers and no more. You know that.

I'm too embarrassed.

I can have one of my colleagues do it.

I don't trust anyone else.

You've boxed me in.

Not me. It's the situation.

So the procedures hovered just over the horizon like cloud shapes, more apparent than real — we see them but cannot approach. Well, they never did get done. Darkness remained without hope of a single torch.

The calls slowed down, then picked up. The procedures stopped getting scheduled. Darkness continued and beat against the dining room window. And Chacon herself was unchanged.

Housing was no different.

Weight was no different.

Tendency to hang around my office for hours talking to whoever was there was no different.

General state of misery, no different.

As best I could tell, I'd had no positive effect whatsoever.

Jonathan Ungar, she said. You know, he's one of your colleagues.

Yeah?

I mean, you refer patients to each other?

Sometimes.

There's something about him you don't know.

I'm sure.

No, Jon and me, I mean.

Question is, Chacon, do I really *want* to know.

It's nothing bad. He was a resident at the time, pretty unhappy about things. We had conversations.

Lots of people do.

He was pretty unhappy, and we actually ended up lying beside each other one night, most of the night. There was no sex or anything...

Chacon, I don't need to know this.

... no sex at all. Sex for me had become such a horrible thing. That's why as an escort I didn't have sex with the men, well, mostly, well, I mean, not at all.

And hearing this against my will, I wondered if this was the same quality of speaking that made incredible things seem plausible, that tonal certainty that suffused the lie that made it all plausible for her and with such ease to morph from, for example, voluntary file clerk to Office Manager Without Pay.

How much truth does it take to feed the morph?

I don't think I heard that, I said.

Heard what?

What you said about Jon.

I think he's pretty uneasy about that.

No comment.

And I filed that item away along with all the snippets I received and initially distrusted from my staff, who spoke with eyebrows raised, saying Chacon was implying things around the office that suggested a kind of relationship between *us*, the treacherous kind of implications that, if honored by a response, seem to take on merit.

And the stack of memorabilia got a voice and began talking to me with line breaks.

Mythology, it said.
Epic.
Terrors and distortions.
Images and holograms slipped between the pages.

So I looked one day

and there were images of a woman and child. That would be the
   sister.
X-ray report of a deformity of the right hip, unclear whether or not
   it was trauma . . .
A general letter from Dr. Hoder asking if there is something some-
   one can do for this patient.
A book of her father's poems dedicated to all those who made it
   possible "for me to change from humanist to misanthrope."
Notebooks filled with accounts of warnings from her parents not to
   tell "David" anything about them or they would destroy her.
The medical name she had found for her condition: Munchausen's
   Syndrome by Proxy.
Letters from her father late in life always ending with I LOVE YOU
   written in giant red letters, the final one containing a prayer that
   God take him in exchange for healing her.
Reconciliation is impossible, he had said, except through letters
   written about good things.
A self-portrait of her naked with roses in hand, pills on the floor,
   the sketch entitled "No, no, no."

She'd put her life and her tragedy in my hands.

How much larger her burden than anything I could have imagined.

The artifacts in my drawer swelled and groaned. The stack took for itself a name, and that name was The Museum of Chacon History. There was a black wooden statue of a sitting chieftain the king of Monrovia gave her father when he was some kind of trader along the coast of Africa.

I have some end tables with Italian marble tops, she said. Do you want them?

When do we get started on the book? she asked. We *are* going to write the book together, aren't we? My life is a story that *has* to be told. Something must come of this. That's why we came together after all this time, isn't it?

You're writing a book with Chacon? my staff wanted to know.

Not that I know of, I said. It was an answer that sounded both true and false, an answer meant to establish reluctance, innocence, independence, something to separate me from the suck of the whirlpool around her and the ruthless posture of advantage taking that seemed so much a part of it. Yet the story was there, throbbing like a hidden heart.

Then she told me . . .

. . . how her father would sneak into her bedroom at night . . .

I would hear his footsteps coming down the hall, hear the floor creak under his weight. Hear the rasp of his hand against the wallpaper as he approached the door. I knew every click and squeak of hinge, every groan of threshold, every rustle of bedclothes coming undone. It was only me. No one else. My sister . . . was spared. She doesn't understand. That's why she won't speak to me. That's why she refuses to believe. She's the favorite and got all the money because she defends him and rejects anything sordid about my father and me.

My father loved me.

How can you say that?

He loved me! He came to my bed anytime he wanted. And I loved him and I . . . I hated *me*. That's just how it was. And I knew I made him do it. It was I who desired *him*. I who allowed myself to be attractive enough to lure him. How could it have been otherwise? How could he have been so awful? He was a famous man.

Each morning Mother gave me enemas to clean me out, to make me pure. She never said anything about it, but I could tell what she was doing and I knew — oh yes — I knew she knew about everything.

Realization crept over my skin like a dirty disease, a sudden rash of scabies snipping and sniggling and burrowing in. Something seized inside me. This was the tragedy she wore like a blue tattoo. This was the corruption of her body and her struggle to love and punish. This was why, all this time, I could not cast her out. It was not her fault.

On his deathbed I asked him why, she said, why did you do this to me?

God gave you to me, he said.

What do you mean?

I prayed and prayed for a son. He didn't give me a son. Instead he gave me you. You were his apology. His gift. My payment for never getting a son.

I tried to imagine a child, lying in bed with all the insecurities and needs a child has, wanting to expect from her father protection, honor, something just to make the night go right, having instead to expect that her father would intrude upon her repeatedly, invading her safety, her body. Invading the life she hoped later to lead.

By day she was the child who respected her father, learned from her father, lingered under the protective arc of her father's care and trust . . . and by night . . . there was no recourse. Her mother refused the idea, washing the essence of it away in the foamy flux of enema after enema after enema . . . after . . . enema . . .

You belong to me, he said. I will do as I wish.

And I saw a child in her bed surrounded by her own emotions, hope, shame, love, fear. When I was that age, shivering in the cold aftermath of a nightmare, I would call for my mother. She would come to me, rub my back, sing to me, and by grace restore me once again to the compensated world.

Chacon's father *was* the nightmare, not the poultice but the perpetrator. Not the intruder outside but the one within ordained by God.

Chacon and the image of Chacon have slowly disappeared. The burden was too great. Her story too large. It had revealed itself slowly, the way large things must come in small pieces announcing the next astonishment when the soul has made room for the last, rising like a dark moon over a river of sorrow.

Then only the little flashes of insanity, the little yelps and barks that bounce off the side of our comfortable walls, then nothing. The workup never got done, housing never solved, the water in her apartment never stopped. The stack of memorabilia swelled and reached its arc, the notes it carried from the center of a perpetual breakdown seething with voices and mumbles, sorrows and hopes, searching for a vague architecture of love.

Ready for Anything

Okay, so I'm ready for anything, and I recognize the feeling, that suspension of sound and motion when your brain knows something big is on the way.

I drive the Tahoe–Truckee highway, my right arm cradled across my lap, my left hand doing the work, turning the ignition, shifting gears, releasing the brake, now driving the car behind a line of cars possibly also headed to find out something important. I am not impatient, even when realizing I am impaired and alone, not as disturbed as perhaps I should be. In the unhurried moments between things I ponder how my feeling is the opposite of worry. Worry is all about *imagined* danger. When real danger comes a new mechanism takes over, as if under the vapors of the daily anxieties there is hidden this playing field of the serious. Bizarre. Maybe what is to come will also be bizarre.

Behind me in their ski lessons are my sons, one skiing, one waiting, while my wife, realizing she will be with one or the other the rest of the day, has placed her skis and her boots in the back of the car I am driving, where they rattle against each whatever, jibe and juke over the bouncy ice chunks in the road.

Have you had your holiday injury yet?

I shift in my seat. I'm earning a reputation I'd rather not have, this annual December-January ski injury of mine, which now is a flash of anticipation in the eyes of my patients as we approach that time of year, I, resolving that I should act my age and consider, well, safety, for example, ever hereafter leaving my children's ski lessons to the experts. Hold my hand, he said on the icy slope. Skis crossed, and when the stun that got the undivided attention of every cell in my body had faded, there was a crackling feeling every time I moved my right shoulder.

Now as I sit in this slow-moving car I just know the damn thing is broken. And I just know I have not seen the worst of this. On my strangely leisurely way to the Forrest General ER, not in very much pain but knowing more is on its way, I am wondering what the prehistoric guys did to ride this kind of stuff out. There will be bleeding into the joint. It might as well be kerosene the way blood sets up trouble in there. Maybe not knowing too many details would be better.

The smell of Fritos wafts toward me. By now I have met the Pollyanna at the triage desk, the courteous male nurse who took my probably hell-of-a-lot-higher-than-usual blood pressure, received a paging device that looks like the hyperactive electronic Wheel of Fortune they give you to queue at a fancy restaurant, and gone to watch videos of downhill wipeouts along with all the other ski-slope victims in the waiting room.

A little girl maybe six years old in a red ski outfit is the culprit munching the Fritos. The aroma is not appetizing. Strangely, the scene makes me think of Hollywood.

Have you had your holiday injury yet? That would be Gina, my massage therapist, asking. That was last week. This was the first time she had seen me not injured in a long time. I must be losing my touch.

The girl in the red jacket doesn't appear injured, but she's with someone who is — a snowboard guy, right hand bandaged. Family all around. And I thought, Why bring my family here to just wait and wait while I wait and wait to find out what we need to know? Let them ski. Sorry, I had said to Duston, beating him to the apology and the remorse.

Funny how the body goes quiet like this — just calm all over, waiting for the disordered part to come back in line, the wound to organize itself. I am getting a view usually I get secondhand, the silk purse in this case fresh appreciation for what my patients go through. My throat feels relaxed, head a little woozy, thoughts narrow. My metabolism has dimmed its lights.

Peter, you ready?

We are poised at the mouth of the X-ray suite. And I don't know if it's to be my X-ray or someone else's.

We'll take the layers off one at a time, she said, good side first. Tight, but easier than I thought, and my good sweater did not have to be cut in pieces off my body after all. Professionals here.

My eyes burn from the sunblock I put on with religious fervor and I don't need now but lingers anyway, doing its duty.

On the road I had wondered about the orthopedist. I told my wife this is the kind of thing, not knowing what kind of thing it was, that sometimes needs surgery. Belzer. That was the name of the shoulder guy in San Francisco. Arrangements of time rise before me — would I go back to pick them up before surgery, before driving back to San Francisco, but how would we check out of the motel . . . ?

Might need surgery. Marvelous how easy the words come, I who have not had surgery since I was a little boy, who has not taken a pain reliever in all adulthood, and who has issues about going under. I had blithely said the words without flinching. And now, driving the road to the possibility of surgery, closer mile by mile, I have not gotten all heated up about it, and I even visualized easily the going under, as if fear has no ace to play in the presence of the *real* deal.

Shivering now, I am draped in a light gown, sitting in the white light of the X-ray room. The attendant, Peter, having shrugged his shoulders as I came in as if to say, Nobody told me about this one, has left me sitting here, quivering partly from what the body does when it is harmed, partly because the temperature seems to be dropping as I wait with nothing to contain my warmth, my broken piece of body floating in the soup of what was, until today, an intact working ball-and-socket joint, waiting for this marvelous ray of intelligence to land upon it and disclose its new name.

The tech peeks around the corner behind the venetian blinds, says something I don't understand, and disappears.

Put your back to the plate. Ah, the tech is back.

I size him up. How are you doing? I ask.

He is thrown off by my question. Okay, he says, trying to recover. How are you?

It's a question he probably wished he hadn't asked.

Right shoulder?

Right shoulder.

I need a pelvis and a chest. That was the shout that bounced off the hard tile walls, careening in from the next room. Then the radiologist needs to see her films right away, it said.

Somebody sicker than I am, I thought. Hope she's okay.

I have to get you to lean over...

He's taking the overhead shot now, and as I feel the click of something over something else that shouldn't be clicking around like that, my arm splays out in precisely the position I have been working hard to avoid. I'm visualizing a free part of me floating around in there. A tightness binds the wing-blade tip as if a hand of muscle holds the tender pieces in check.

I'll come and tell you the results, he said as I slipped back in bed, in the gurney, that is, my new chaise longue.

Thank you.

One o'clock. The boys are through with their lessons now, and I don't know anything. I should call even so.

No service — probably shouldn't call from here anyway.

An orderly passes. Cell phones all right here?

I'll check... No, they're not.

Didn't take long to find that out. Strange, the not knowing that separates me from my family right now. Just as well. Nothing to say.

And what about that tingling in my fingers right after the accident that I forgot to tell anyone about but now remember that I thought was just the cold? Mostly gone. Right side tingling gone long ago. Left side fading. I must have cranked my neck pretty good, kinked my spinal cord, pinched a few nerves as they left the depot to steam along the train tracks down to my hands.

Well, nothing's fallen off, I hear from the next bed. They're going to X-ray it. Just the tailbone . . .

This place is busy. Must be that ice on the slopes this morning. That's what started the fear in my son in the first place. Damn smart idea sometimes, fear.

The ER doctor is motoring toward the young lady directly across from me a clacking, jangling, full-scale model of the human skeleton. It was the woman he had asked just a mite ago, What happened to you? even though I could tell from way over here. Must be a standard opening here in ski country.

It's a fracture of T3, he says, pointing to the spot on the human form, naked of everything but bones. Some of these fractures are unstable, he says, but this one looks pretty good.

I am relieved all the way over here.

The fracture is normally in the body of the vertebra, he says. Yours is crunched down to about half its height. You've lost volume, but there are still two millimeters or so before it hits the spinal cord.

The young man standing over her I remember from the triage desk. He was on the phone saying, X-rays done, but we don't know anything yet. He seemed confident and efficient. Not worried.

We're going to admit you and take care of you, the doctor was saying.

Her young man, his finger in the hole of the skeleton's spinal column, asked about that two-millimeter stuff.

There's a smudge on the sheet where I put my foot. My shoulder is beginning to freeze.

Gina will be amused.

The young man is bringing a cup with a straw.

What happened to you?

I was helping my son . . .

It was the doctor speaking. Let me show you what you've done. He flashes his films. You've got a tear of the acromioclavicular ligament. A shoulder separation. Just a sling and some pain meds, and in a few weeks you'll be okay.

So the clicking I was feeling was the unrestrained ball of the shoulder head dislocating itself over and over, bone rattling against bone like liar's dice.

Should I tell you about this? he asks.

Tell all, I say.

There are three grades of tear, first degree, second degree, and completely torn in two. The last requires surgery. You're probably somewhere between one and two.

Lucky.

Could have been worse. But we can see the separation. It's pretty wide. Still, it should do with a sling and a little time.

And I felt a shift in my position, though my position had not moved. In the previous moment I was one of the herd of the unfortunate awaiting surgery or admission or . . . and I had rehearsed the whole thing, the Big Casino, anesthesia, intubation, repair. I had traveled all those directions a considerable distance and returned, trying out my steps, making channels open into the unknown like breath advancing along a narrow balloon, pressing apart the sticky sides, channeling into the uninflated those ominous pathways I'd never wanted to open but did.

Really beautiful, the EMT was saying to the semiconscious boy on the stretcher. Good pulse, he said, as if the pulse were the only important thing — we're going to get you taken care of.

And I am no longer down that channel. How easily we count ourselves among the lost, how easily we dispense with fear when it arises out of the imagination. I am in my sling on the way to my car. Sitting in the driver's seat before I begin the curiously conscious task of driving, I will call my wife. Fantastic, she will say, the boys were just asking about you. And then I will call Kate, who had reached me just as I was gingerly sliding into the car to ask about the biopsy report on her ulcer. Are you all right? she had said, sensing the back story to my voice. I think I just broke my shoulder, I said.

I will ease her worries.

And then, reaching my left hand over the steering column to turn the key, I will shift gears, release the brake, and start driving.

I might even listen to a little salsa music on the way.

A Critical Distance

She's off service, the nurse said.

Off service?

Yeah.

What do you mean, off service?

She's no longer the attending physician. She's rotated to another service.

I would like to talk to her.

It won't do any good. She's passed your wife along to the next attending.

Does that mean she's not available?

The October attending is on service now.

Who is the October attending?

She's the attending that comes in October.

Emily had come to the Teaching Hospital to have her baby. Her thinking was there was a good chance this might be a complicated pregnancy, possibly like the first, and she wanted to be in the best of hands.

Her first child, a girl, was taken from her warm innerspace two months early, ushered into the world prematurely under the slow glow of that swelling tempest known as toxemia of pregnancy that, once anchoring itself upon the horizon, moves closer without any possibility of delay.

She bloated. She got heavy. Her kidneys leaked like sieves. She puffed up like a poisoned pup. It was not pretty.

Her husband, a doctor, thought she was courageous, maybe

even crazy, to try a second pregnancy. Thrilled and at the same time terrorized, he thought the choice to go to the university was just right. Last time she'd started with a midwife, a decision in which he indulged her, and she ended up smack dab in the local hospital. This new decision was, in his view, stepping up to the major leagues.

This pregnancy, as was the first, was an IVF pregnancy, egg donation — the arduous process of desire and invasion after the roller-coaster ride of wanting children late in life, never imagining the two of them could not send forward into the universe the characteristics of each other they loved. First came sorrow, then fragile hope as her own eggs, pushed and prodded and pummeled, swelled and died. Then came despair, whipped about, as they were, like a fly on a casting line — one minute drifting, the next ripped through the trembling air as their attempts fluttered and failed.

So they made one with another woman's egg.

The first child, barely four and a half pounds, spent ten days in the ICU, hovering on the edge of existence, breathing, not breathing. Once home they watched her breathe for six months before they were able to get a full night's sleep.

Now another series of injections in her rump and simultaneously in the rump of the "egg mother," hormones flowing into the system in order to synchronize their yolk cycles, then that remarkable, magical egg harvest, fishing spheres like small solar systems from the galaxy of her ovaries, fertilization in a petri dish, incubation under a watchful microscope, cell division, the elegantly timed beginnings at the periphery of life to shape that rollup of cells that would organize themselves into the blastocyst, and then, at just the right moment, implantation . . .

Then hope, that fickle old friend.

Six weeks later she feels a sudden sharp pain in her right lower belly, and over the phone her husband knows what it is. An errant zygote, a swelling fetus, misplaced perhaps by a swish of the injection that placed it there, propelled beyond the uterus to the Fallopian tube, where it grew a stunted, angular growth, pressing against the bulbous tube, where it would, if not tended, burst and do in both child and mother.

911. Ambulance ride. Sonogram — one heart beating in the soft nest of uterus, another, smaller, hiccupping from the confinement of the tube. Midnight surgery. Spinal anesthesia, she chose, so as not to chemically disturb the child in the uterus, which meant she was wide awake.

The pain you feel is supposed to be there, the doctor said.

Brilliant, she thought. That separates away the fear.

Then home again.

a blue hush
and then a piece
of sky

in between
pulse and dissolve
like cream
in my coffee

my newspaper
open
conversation
or none
one seed in humus
the other
stone

how quiet
the chatter of heartbeat
how small

the spark so quick
it never started

everything is
as it was
you lie sleeping

I sit in a chair

a quiet breath
in the room

Block Island had sounded really good. Sand, sea, but mostly time and its altered state of motion when it moves at the seashore. Reservations made long ago. East Coast relatives to meet them there, coming and going into a pause with no schedule.

The bags were stacked by the door. Taxi service arranged — early morning pickup to the shuttle. Then the plane.

She was approaching seven months. And there were little, recognizable alterations that by themselves had no significance at all — a little bloating, some headaches, slowed urination. Taken separately they mean nothing; together they built the materials and structures of that stealthy old problem. If it *was* toxemia again, she'd not receive the shots, the Decadron to hasten the infant's air sacks toward maturity. Less chance, that way, of suffocation by lungs that will not work. Thirty-two weeks was the daughter's arrival. It was thirty-one weeks now, and *it* was beginning to show.

Well, why couldn't I deliver on the East Coast if I get in trouble? Yes, but . . .

I want to go, she said. We'll be all right.

There is a special quality of anxiety that comes when you're about to distance yourself from the help you need, when the signs of the need are already rising off the surface of the earth like a dust devil. Dread permeated his body. He didn't sleep. He started taking her blood pressure. The diastolic was rising, 88, 92, now 98, a clear sign. It added to his distress. If it added to hers, she didn't show it. She was determined.

The taxi came, and in it piled the pregnant couple, their daughter, and all their hopeful baggage.

At the shuttle bus pickup, sitting next to them on his way to lecture at a conference in Tokyo, was the chief of obstetrics and gynecology at her husband's hospital. It might have been the fact that he raised his eyebrows in a convincing manner. It might have been one more blood pressure reading where she sat on the bench — but the shuttle left, and they took the taxi back home. Next day she was in the hospital.

The university hospital.

Who's your doctor? they asked at admissions.

She said the name.

The clerk looked away for what seemed like a long time, all the while clicking and shuffling her mouse over and over.

No, she finally said. It's going to be Dr. ——.

That's not my doctor.

It's the doctor on service, honey. She's going to be your doctor in the hospital.

I never met her. She's not my doctor.

It's whoever the attending is on service. That's your doctor. Clinic doctors only do outpatient work.

Then the wrist band, the IV, the intern, the resident, the medical student, asking the same questions and writing the same notes in the chart . . . and her headache deepened, blood pressure lifted. They started a drip of magnesium sulfate.

A few hours later the chief resident came in and said they planned to induce her.

What does that mean?

To give you hormones that make your uterus contract, make you go into labor.

Why do that? Don't we have to do a C-section like was done before? And do it soon?

We'd like to try induction first.

Then the first-year resident came in and said they were thinking about doing a C-section.

Then the second-year resident came in and said that induction was too dangerous.

The nurse came in and hung the Ptocin. She told her that it was the hormone that would make her uterus contract.

Is that induction?

That's induction, she said, and started hooking monitor leads to the mother and child.

What's that for?

To watch for danger signs.

Cramps, then nausea, then the out-of-touch-with-reality feeling that she couldn't describe but made night turn into day and then the other side of night without the conscious passing of hours. Time was immobile, sideways, disconnected from the events of the day, which went on happening without pattern or plan.

Her husband asked to speak to the attending.

She's on rounds.

I want to speak with her.

We'll page her.

No one came.

Meanwhile, the drip went on dripping.

So he went out to the nursing station and inquired. Probably only because he was a doctor, someone gestured in the direction of the residents' room, where the doctors were holding rounds. He went in, asked for the attending, who turned to him and kindly —patronizingly, he thought—explained that they didn't do C-sections unless induction had failed.

But she's already had a C-section. Doesn't that mean she will most likely need another? And what about the length of time she had to stay in this toxic state with blood pressure rising . . . wasn't that dangerous?

We think she can deliver.

There was nothing to do but wait.

He made camp in her room, the Naugahyde sofa his perch and his bed. She drifted in a painful soup of disorientation and nausea. The baby wasn't moving. The contractions were not propelling the womb or its cargo. The hours ticked uncounted.

You can tell from her face
she floats above her body
while they make her body do

what they want it to — she steps aside
for the taking over —
the steering wheel, the driving instructor —

How unlike she thought it would be
this is, hovering between consciousness
and the conscious will to choose.

Hallelujah, after all, for Fentanyl, for the lack
of feeling it gives as the body motors
through delivery, or doesn't, that sweet episode

trapped in its unraveling nest,
a silver rim of light opening
between mother and child.

Next shift, a new nurse. Tough cookie. For sure she pumped iron daily to maintain her buff, muscular form, her close-cropped hair leaving space to appreciate the accented definition of the muscles in her neck and upper back as she bent over her charge with clean, efficient motions.

How are you doing?

It was a question that had no answer but the answer given out of falsehood and courtesy.

They talked about the induction thing.

My other doctor would have had that baby out of there by

now. And I could be over this. Maybe that would have been better.

The nurse was a team player. No sympathy for that other point of view was remotely visible in the flashing of her eyes. Take your medicine and let the decisions be made by those with better abilities to make them.

Has the magnesium dose increased?
No. And it was

the isolated no, the no
of a mother or a schoolmarm.

It lay over the air between nurse and patient
like a moth on swamp risings —

the nurse's perspective jostling against
the patient's perspective, perturbation among ideas

how to go about a labor
and delivery — the seasons

of pain and joy grown ordinary
as clichés. I know

what my other OB would do, she said.
He'd say let's get that baby

out of there right now — the headache speaking,
the lover and the morphine speaking,

in the room waves the red plume of overresponse
and the wisdom of underresponse as the days

slow down to the I-can't-seem-to-get-anything-done
kind of days, where spaces fall back in

between the numerals of the day
and you notice again as you walk how light spills

on the sidewalk out from cafes
where people clink their glasses

and dishes on your way back from dinner to the hospital
where you will sleep better than you thought you would

on the half-sized, some-kind-of-slippery-material
sofa with the one thermal blanket

and where in the two slow hours of morning
you will watch her finally sleep.

Friday afternoon, thirty-six hours later, and she was dwindling like the last flicker of an oil lamp.

I'm not in control here, she said. It's terrifying. What's worse is that I don't even know who to talk to. I guess that would be the attending, but the attending never comes. Is it arrogance? Are they afraid of me? Is this just some unfortunate accident of complexity, too many people on the team? No one stepping up to the plate?

I know there are some things you can't control, she said. But it would help to feel like you have someone to *accompany* you. It's like there is this critical distance they have placed between doctor and patient. I can't see them, I can't see the decisions they are making about me as if I'm some kind of puppet. It's puppet-string medicine.

He went out to find the attending.

That's when he learned it was now the October attending.

I need to speak to him.

Her.

Okay, her. I need to speak to her right away.

We'll page her.

The C-section was planned for two P.M.

At five P.M. they wheeled her into the room.

Her husband was relieved that relief was finally in sight before the C-section was even begun, before the baby was known to be a boy or a girl or to be strong or to be vulnerable or even in one piece after all these chemicals and toxins and the suffering through the long and sideways hours together — before knowing all that, just to know a positive action, some kind of action, was being taken.

He sat on a stool at the head of her gurney as the anesthesiology resident sat her up and began to insert the needle into her spinal column, seeking the exact place to give the perfect level of relief she needed to do this thing. And then he laid her back down again.

The surgeon raised the scalpel, testing the surface of the abdomen for the numbness she expected.

Owwwww!

Up again and another attempt to place the needle.

Down again.

Owwww!

Up again, down again, up again. An hour passed. The surgeon grabbed the anesthesia attending, who had been standing there all this time watching, and yanked him out of the room.

When they returned the anesthesia attending whisked the resident aside and took over. Five minutes later the surgery began.

It was a boy.

They didn't even let her hold him. Maybe they "showed" him to her, maybe not. All she remembered was hearing him cry and feeling reassured.

Then the hemorrhaging began. It came as a large clot all at once when she rose to try, for the first time, to walk to the bathroom. Then brighter blood. Lots and lots. Then she fainted.

Ptocin, they said, and brought some.

A huge cramp followed, but the bleeding didn't stop.

The resident, without anesthesia or sedation and without announcing what she was doing, pushed her hand against the grain of the birth canal, which had never been used as a birth canal, and ripped clot and debris from the inside of the uterus.

The cry that came from her lips was ancient, filled with every woman's pain and anguish, every woman's rage at the breach at the door of her body that would-not-did-not-could-not stop even when it was supposed to stop, and her wail, echoing down the corridors of the Teaching Hospital, was heard by everyone.

Three in the morning. She had bled her hematocrit down to a dangerous 20 percent. She had lost half her blood. The new attending told her it would take maybe a couple of months for her own bone marrow to replace the lost blood, but you'll do all right, she said. You're young enough.

And Emily could not sleep. Tied into the electrical space above her bed, she could not drop down to the soft blanket of sleep. Each little relaxation, shot through by a nervous charge, alerted her to some new or imagined threat.

Finally, when the rumble from a thousand nerve endings settled to a flickering sizzle over the surface of her body, she could, at last, sink into the deepening trough of her bed.

Five-thirty A.M. that was. She drifted as if drifting had been forgotten, dropping like silt into the healing arms of sleep . . .

Wake up, wake up!

Her eyes rolled toward light, but the lids would not open. She raised her brow, and still they stayed closed. With her hands she lifted them by their lashes and forced them to open to the clock resting on the bedside table. 5:53 A.M., it said. She had been asleep less than thirty minutes.

What emergency, she thought.

Her eyes wobbled to see. There standing over her was the medical student.

What, what is . . . ?

She was not able to finish.

So. Have you nursed your baby yet? the medical student asked, jovially.

Oh. Well, I haven't even seen my baby yet, she said.

I need to ask you a question, said the medical student.

Question?

Yes, I have rounds in a little while, and I need to know what form of birth control you plan to use when you go home.

Emily was without words. And before they might form themselves out of the mists of confusion she found herself groping for meaning.

Then it came to her. They weren't there to help her. Not to help her so much as they were there to do their jobs. The medical student's job was to appear knowledgeable about the patient on rounds. The medical student didn't know the information she thought she might need to know, so, rather than fishing it out of the chart, she just woke up the patient.

It had come to that.

The medical student was the eye of the cone that opened back to the attending deciding to do induction because it was the academic thing to do, the discrepancies in the mouths of the multiple faces coming into her room, the anesthesia attending allowing the resident with the amateur hands too much time . . . *They'd paid more attention to their rounds than to their patient.*

And now, after all, the medical student had decided to wake up the exhausted patient rather than look bad on rounds.

If Emily had within her the energy to scream, she would have . . . but she'd done that. The scream was out of her now, and there was nothing but cold reality to take its place.

She fixed the medical student with her unsteady eyes.

Read the chart, she said. I'm infertile.

The medical student slinked out, but the damage was done. Emily was awake now, unable by ability or trick to find a new way to sleep again, caught between rage and the jazz beyond rage, unable to lay her soul back down inside the frame of the body, nor would she be, until she wheeled herself out of the hospital, out of town, out of the reach of doctors to her own safe bed.

Yet she didn't sleep until she had slept awhile, like the work you have to do before the work you need to do. Then she slept deeply, as if it was the medicinal ooze out of which she could be reborn into the world, the poisons leeching slowly from her body, the body reclaiming itself.

It was three days before she saw her son.

For a week she rose only to pee off a pound or two and then sink into the prow of her bed, down to where the unholy sins in her body, molecule by molecule, would slide slowly from her.

And the child lay apart from her in its own bed, a distance away in the Intensive Care Unit, surrounded by what could not be loved but needed to be there, moving his body slowly toward existence, the son and the mother rising separately and together into the world.

The Way We Know
What We Know

Every time I bring up anxiety, she said, my therapist says it's my past issues coming up.

Christine is about forty, thin, somewhat muscular in the manner of someone who has exercised a lot or lived awhile in the wilderness. She holds a sheet of paper in her hands and a pen with which she occasionally takes notes, nodding her head, as if doing so etched the words more strongly onto the page, letter by letter, securing for them both place and rhythm.

Past issues, she said. I don't think I have any. Actually, I had a very *good* childhood. So then my therapist tells me I'm fighting her. Am I fighting her?

Christine has a degree in literary criticism from Brown University. Having no illusions that her training would produce a secure career for her, she drifted off into physical fitness, became a tour guide on kayaking trips, could do a rollover and come up smiling. When her thyroid failed she changed her diet, took herbs, exercised harder, and finally consented to taking a little synthetic thyroid hormone. The sluggishness she had felt in her well-toned legs and arms improved. Her depression improved. Yet she was hard to regulate. Her lab results revealed a slow drift, this way and that, that required close attention, changing ever so slightly the micrograms of vital hormone she required.

She experienced long periods of depression, pushing against her like a giant wave that never seemed willing to crest and fall.

She questioned herself. She doubted her life. She worried she might be *responsible* for her condition.

I reminded her of the electrochemical soup of the brain, how transmitters worked, how the little sparkles of communication depend upon chemistry to keep us lit up. I recalled a time in the history of medicine before we had lab tests to help us, when sanatoriums were jammed with unrecognized hypothyroid patients. Myxedema Madness, they called it. Dropping a little thyroid pill in the right teacup cured many a psychosis.

Maybe you need a new psychologist, I said.

Do you think so?

Mixed in her question was the hope of salvation from these forced reentries into the past but also a little self-doubt over the possibility she might be mistaken about the nil effect of her history. A struggle played out between reason and feeling.

I suppose there is a possibility that I'm fighting against it, she went on, because I *am* afraid at some level.

What does your heart say?

What do you mean?

Well, it sounds like you're approaching this intellectually. The intellect will focus on the possibility, no matter how remote, that something *might* be wrong. That leads to distortion, blockage. The heart is rarely confused. It doesn't care for details, just lands on what it wants.

During all this time she had been sitting with her hands folded over her comfort object, the sheet of paper resting like a peripheral brain on her lap, her body inert but for the narrow oscillations of her chin as she spoke. Now suddenly she leaned back, as if to recoil from a gust of strong wind.

A smile ticked and struggled at the corner of her mouth.

I guess "what do you *feel*" is the question, I said. That's the way we know what we know.

She remained silent.

You can trust what you feel. My guess is that if you do not believe there is profit to be had from excavating the past, then you're probably right. After all, you have good reason to be depressed, biochemical reasons. And as you know, depression is often accompanied by anxiety.

How can I be sure?

Ah, certainty. It was the brain speaking, wanting to be convinced beyond a shadow of a doubt. Pesky brain. Persistent brain.

I needed something more than reason to communicate. Something that bypassed the brain directly to the heart.

Do you know "The Soft Animal of the Body"? I said.

Now she looked really confused.

It's from a poem by Mary Oliver called "Wild Geese."

I don't know it.

During recent months I had typed into my computer, under the file name "Poems for the Time Capsule," a few poems capable of generating strong shifts in thinking, chosen partly for their beauty but perhaps mostly for the effect they had on me personally, moving foundations, opening new ideas. I had been following the wisdom of Galway Kinnell, who said that if we memorize, we incorporate more deeply into our consciousness. All the way down to the genome — so I imagined. I printed out a few of these and on my commute to work memorized them. Now was the occasion to speak one.

So I did.

You do not have to be good.
You do not have to walk on your knees
for a hundred miles through the desert, repenting.
You only have to let the soft animal of your body
love what it loves.
Tell me about despair, yours, and I will tell you mine.
Meanwhile the world goes on.
Meanwhile the sun and the clear pebbles of the rain

are moving across the landscapes,
over the prairies and the deep trees,
the mountains and the rivers.
Meanwhile the wild geese, high in the clean blue air,
are heading home again.
Whoever you are, no matter how lonely,
the world offers itself to your imagination,
calls to you like the wild geese, harsh and exciting —
over and over announcing your place
in the family of things.

I noticed that at the end of each phrase it was her body that responded, beginning in the manner of rousing itself to light or music and then loosening a little about the shoulders and knees, allowing a gesture of the open palm, the drifting arm off to one side, the arc of a smile breaking.

When the poem finished she nodded and bowed her head.

Thank you, she said.

Thank you, Mary Oliver, I said. For I could see how the poem, in ways I could not, had touched something in her, as if it had entered the rhythms of her body in a manner only known to the body.

What she was thinking I could not say and would not ask. It would be different from what I was thinking, particular to what she only might think. That's how poetry works, speaking to us in our own particular language.

Nothing more to say about that.

I'll recheck your thyroid in two months, okay?

She nodded and rose from her chair. Put away her little piece of paper and started for the door. And all the while I'd thought it was for *my* benefit I'd memorized those poems.

As we walked toward the appointment desk I realized that to talk about an idea and to feel an idea are two different things. Presented with the beauty of words that sing alongside each other, the idea may find its path to the heart. Knowledge, without the consent of the heart, changes little.

Christine stopped by the front desk to make her new appointment. I heard her talking about poetry to my patients who were waiting there. Somehow, the way she spoke, my patients were not astonished.

She was done with her visit.

She was on her way to the bookstore.

Third Opinion

Maybe you know why I'm here, she said.

I did know. This morning she didn't have an appointment. This afternoon she did, less a testimony to the flexibility of our office than to her dogged British persistence.

I find myself in somewhat difficult circumstances, she said.

I know, I said.

You know?

I just talked to Dr. Hoskins.

I've known Hoskins forever, even before the time he left the university to go into the private practice of obstetrics and gynecology. It used to be that patients frequently went back and forth between us, less of that over the years. I might never have met this man.

David, he said in a tone of voice more familiar than the institutional distance our practices might have suggested. David, what are we going to do with Edith?

Already Edith had cut her path with me. Practically the first thing she said was, I don't put much stock in medicines. That was the general tone of things. Therefore, when it came to any new medical event there was always exceeding scrutiny, especially when it came to medicines or procedures.

I know the situation, I told her.

She looked at me as if to say, No matter what you think you know, you won't know it *correctly* until you are informed by me.

As you may know, she said — and she said it in a way that made me realize how Southern drawls could be generated from the British capacity to bend the sly turn of pivotal words — I have a son in New York. And you were exactly right when you said there would be opinions about this.

I didn't remember commenting. Perhaps she was remembering a general tendency of mine from a previous time. Perhaps she was just pointing out a collegiality of thought.

He put me in touch with a very respectable gynecologist there who said you treat a seventy-two-year-old woman the same way you treat a thirty-five year old . . . you go after it aggressively.

I was remembering what Hoskins said. Look, David, he said. You don't want to put an old lady through all that oncology crap. You want to just get in there, get it out, and go home . . .

Edith was going on in her deliberate and resonant voice. He says you do this . . . what do you call it. And she pointed one finger repeatedly in a stabbing motion at her belly button.

Laparoscopy.

. . . laparoscopy, laparosco-pic-ally, or whatever, and do a good . . . *thorough* — the stress on the word came with both her voice and the high, arched lift of an eyebrow — *search*.

I thought of her writerly manner with words and of the novel she'd written for children, a copy of which I had at home but had not read. I must read this, I thought.

What do *you* think?

I had been drifting along in the relaxing motions of words and accents, and her abrupt shift had a little shock built into it. I like shock. It's necessary at times to get at the root of things.

That's why I'm here, she added, seeing me pause and briefly mute.

You need another opinion, I said.

I've got one, she said. It's you.

Then you need a third.

If she could be direct, so could I. Besides, it saves time and spares us the numbing hesitations of courtesy.

That's what I thought, she said.

And I have just the person, I said, a gynecological oncologist.

That's it, she said, snapping her fingers and becoming suddenly animated. That's it. How do you say it?

Gynecological oncologist.

Yes, that's what my son said. I wasn't sure they made one.

Oh, they do indeed.

But what about Dr. Hoskins?

What about him?

He wants to do surgery on Thursday. Won't that mess up his plans?

His plans. Now a different kind of shock.

A little clarity here, I said. Let's begin at the core.

I leaned over for emphasis.

You're the only important person in this transaction, Edith. Do you know that? We're all, all of us, just here to be in your service.

Doctors in service of the patient?

What a concept.

He won't be offended?

He might. If he is, that's his problem.

She looked unconvinced.

I went on.

This kind of thing happens all the time. I encourage my own patients to get second, even third opinions if they need them. I confess it's a bit easier after being in practice awhile. Maybe it's confidence. Maybe it's the final triumph of generosity. But I've come to understand it's no skin off my nose. Besides, if you don't overdo it, things go better with more brain trust in the tank.

Is this . . . whatever kind of doctor . . . really good?

You'll like her. She's no nonsense. Just like you.

I was feeling uncomfortable in the role of salesman, as if my words hadn't been convincing enough on their own, still unable to accomplish trust. I backed off and dug in.

I wouldn't have recommended her if she wasn't, I said.

Oh, I know that. You've always done well by me. But I have just one more question if I may.

Are you sure?

Would you send your wife to her?

I already did.

Well, she said, and rocked back as if suddenly about to levitate. I must say the cardiologist you sent me to, why, he's . . . I mean you can tell right away . . . he has that sense of . . . authority. I mean in a good way. You can just feel that he has humility and competency.

And I was thinking how gracious it is when humility arrives along with a high competency, confidence, perhaps, of the kind that is comfortable both with what you know and what you don't know and the difference between the two. How much better than arrogance, that sly cover for insecurity.

Now the backstory: this business of her cardiac status and her reluctance to take medications.

She's in atrial fibrillation. Among cardiologists there exists an almost knee-jerk recommendation to give anticoagulants because of the possibility that with all that sludging going on in the disordered, disarticulated atrium a clot might form, which if it does and then gets loose could wreak havoc somewhere — somewhere like the brain, for instance. Gets your attention, all right. I understand. But it's that familiar situation where dire outcome can stir dire measures. So I am always asking, Which is worse?

I remembered my own little burst of atrial fibrillation, brief and notable, and how after just a couple of hours my cardiologist was threatening to hit me with Coumadin. Rat poison. I found myself caught in the wedge between knowledge and the impulse to go against knowledge. I didn't tell him, but I wasn't about to do that. Nor was she, it turns out. Only she carried it a step farther. I converted back to normal rhythm on my own. She did not.

I told her that the rapidity of a beating heart over time sometimes requires digitalis or a beta-blocker to slow it down. Nothing doing, she said. So . . . we are doing just that. Nothing.

The new, lovable cardiologist must have taken all these elements into consideration, including the intuition of the patient. I like that. I thumbed the chart and reread his note. He addressed the issue simply and sharply: he saw no need to change anything before surgery.

He was wonderful, she said.

Because he agrees with us?

She laughed.

Well, I said, he did say you should take a little beta-blocker for a couple of days after surgery.

Sure. But just a couple of days.

I nodded.

Back to the problem of your uterine cancer, I said. And I looked her in the eye.

Yes, she said with a sweep of a hand as if returning to a long letter after a pause. May I ask you *personally* — she strung the word out to its breaking point — to *personally* call the doctor?

No.

Well, you know how it is. I'll probably be given an appointment next October.

Not this time. Your situation won't wait that long. Besides, I know who I'm dealing with here, and she'll get back to me.

I'm afraid to say I don't trust the system.

You're right to be skeptical. Just a bit premature. Let's try the usual way — my receptionist will make the call, and if I need to, I'll jump in.

You will monitor this?

Edith!

This time it was my turn to use the lilting tonalities of the King's English and the fluttering of the eyebrow.

Okay. Okay, she said.

Not entirely satisfied, was she. I knew that. But we were where we needed to be and, having little choice, she relented.

That evening Ruthann called.

Whatcha got, David?

A live one.

Oh boy!

You'll like her. Seventy-two years old and loads of pizzazz.

And uterine cancer, I hear.

The issue is to be aggressive or not to be aggressive.

I did a ninety-four-year-old lady yesterday.

I guess that settles that.

The way to do this is laparoscopically.

I know. We talked about that.

And then be sure to check all the lymph nodes, organs, etc. for metastases.

Sounds right to me.

There's no sense backing off good therapy when it just takes a little longer to do it right.

Yes, indeed! I reflected on my conversation with Hoskins. Come to think of it, he was probably going to do a vaginal hysterectomy. Maybe that meant that he hadn't been trained in laparoscopy and was confining her to his narrow area of competency instead of referring her on. I remembered how violent a "vag hist" is, all that pulling on the uterus to deliver it like a reluctant child through the aging vagina, stretching the round ligament, stretching the ovarian ligaments. Wouldn't that trauma in itself have more of an impact on a seventy-two-year-old woman than a few holes in her belly wall?

Out loud I said that I wasn't comfortable with the possibility of missing something.

Right, Ruthann said.

But Edith may not go for chemo, knowing her, if indeed that comes up.

She may not need it. If she does, we can have that discussion as it makes itself known.

She has to know the variables.

Right.

All this happened on the cusp of my getaway for vacation and a conference. When I returned I called up Ruthann.

How's our lady?

She's good. Maybe going home today. Quite a big lump of tumor.

She had nodes?

I removed them. I don't think they're positive, but we'll see.

How was her attitude?

She seemed happy. She was happy with us. Maybe that could bounce around, shall we say. We had a few complaints, but all went well. And her son was happy. He came out from New York, and he seemed very pleased.

I think you made a hit.

Well, we'll see. You can never rest on your laurels.

Yes, I said, I believe that's it.

Hanna's Volvulus

It's a bit of a mystery. We do it anyway because it seems to work.

I'm explaining the situation we're in to the nurse. Then Hanna chimes in.

The last time we did this it was with the pediatric scope and it wasn't . . . we couldn't get it done.

My recollection was different, but it didn't matter because five minutes later she requested the pediatric scope. I thought you said . . .

Well, I did feel a little better after the pediatric scope, she said.

I began the explanation again. She has a volvulus, I said.

The nurse would know volvulus, a twist of bowel that, like the action that wrings water out of a wash rag, twists the bowel so tight on its pedicel that it shuts down its internal channel. Actually, I've never seen Hanna's volvulus in action. Not a trace, no X-ray, nothing . . . I was bequeathed the diagnosis and the patient when my colleague went north to hang out and do a few endoscopies, as he said. I am performing not my ritual but *his*, I discover, which is to insert a scope periodically into the colon and straighten the twist, imaginary or otherwise, by impaling it on the rapier of the scope. Or, alternatively, to blow enough air in high enough to unravel the colon like a limp balloon.

Pretty mysterious stuff.

Be sure to put enough air in this time, she says.

I will.

Well, last time you didn't think you got all the way.

Yeah, but we did a yeoman's job on that air business.

Explaining all this to the nurse, I feel I may be just giving my current best version of the story. On top of all that, another complication. Now she has a block in the conduction of her heart and practically passed out on my office floor three months ago when her pulse was 36 and blood pressure unattainable, so I got her to a cardiologist and almost as quick as a few minutes later she had a pacemaker in her chest.

Blocked in more places than one, astutely observes the nurse.

Yup. And I am thinking that doing a colonoscopy with a pacemaker in place raises the hair on the back of my neck. It's okay, the cardiologist had said. Still, I'm watching the hiccups on her heart tracing like ticker tape on a morning in October 1929 as I stimulate the vagus nerve with my scope and my blats of air, wondering how safe all this is and if the risk is worth it, especially if this is little more than a fishing expedition.

Now the cardiologists want to put her on blood thinners. I don't like blood thinners. Maybe it's occupational. Bleeding and all that jazz just makes a gastroenterologist go nuts. So that could mean bye-bye colonoscopies. Can't say I'm unhappy about that.

This could be her grand hurrah, I tell my nurse.

She just nods.

And that's not all: she's eighty-one years old, has had asthma and thyroid cancer, is allergic to just about everything in the universe except the sedatives I give her to do this little test, and I'm thinking it's only a matter of time until her immune system blasts away at that too.

Sedatives, I'm thinking, give her sedatives.

I'm not very sedated, she says.

We've just started.

Are you going to be able to get there this time?

Plan to.

Well, last time . . .

I know, I know, but did it work?

How do you mean?

Did you get better?

Well, I don't know.

You told me you got better.

Yeah, I don't want to be doing this thing for nothing.

Me too, buckaroo.

More sedation.

That's something we can agree on.

And I am in now, and I am remembering why I switched to a pediatric scope last time. This sigmoid is a bitch. I withdraw and reposition. No go. I withdraw and torque the scope hard right. I can feel the pressure of the scope against the wall.

How are you doing? I ask.

Just fine.

The lady's tough. But the lady's also eighty-one years old. I do not need to do my first and only perforation on her. I am patient. I wait. Experience tells me that this position will let me slide by if I go really slowly. I increase the pressure. The mucosal surface starts slipping by the lens and then blanches. This means that the pressure against the wall is great enough to squeeze out all the blood. That's what you see in the moment before you end up looking at the pancreas. I stop and release the pressure. All this time I have also been paying attention to her heart rate, which, despite being paced, is slowing down. That means that that viper vagus is rearing its head and spitting nerve hormones through the system. This will mean low blood pressures and other stuff I don't want. I wait. And restart. And wait. Five minutes of this little dance and I pop into the open field of the descending colon. Huzzah!

Diverticulosis, spasm, the usual suspects lie before me. We sail the channel to the transverse colon.

She is weary. Her heart rate is a little irregular, and I count that as three steps closer to atrial fibrillation or something worse. If reaching the ascending colon where the volvulus is supposed to be were the only possible way of benefiting her, I might bide my time, hoping for a clearing in the storm, and then push forward. It's a matter of risk and benefit. I don't quite see the pot of gold at the end of this rainbow, so I drop my payload, a small bomb of air, in the middle of the transverse colon and beat a hasty retreat.

Are you done already?

Yup.

Did you get there?

Yup.

You got all the way to the volvulus.

We got to the vista point.

Vista . . .

Yeah, the good place.

Will I be better?

Yes, indeed.

What she means is, Did I get into the volvulus and straighten it out? I have rendered my strong affirmative. Well, I am on the edge of a lie and I know it, but I don't care. She's going to get better.

And here's the interesting part. The lie is a critical piece. It's that business of expectation and the power it brings. Strong stuff. She will be pleased and comfortable for whatever reason — which reason I may never come to know.

The Case of the
Missing Molecule

The call came in on my cell phone. A 707 number. The microcomputer lodged somewhere in the analysis section of my brain localized the caller to patient, trusted person, someone who should have my number.

Sorry to disturb you, David . . .

I recognized the slow, lilting, Southern drawl. Sounded like summertime under the magnolias.

. . . It's George Tipton, he said.

The rest of the picture flashed in my mind. Brilliant physician and researcher, the kind of guy, like Walter Mountcastle, who would be the laughingstock of the fast-speaking Harvard crowd until he walked away with the best intern award at the end of the year. Southern brilliance. Cloaked and disguised under the sweet sound of slow music.

I got belly pain, he said.

I remembered his long struggle with esophagitis after all those rich meals that as the founder of a multi-billion-dollar research company he was driven to start, which translated into a struggle with acid and stuff. There's a price tag on success.

Same old place? I asked.

No. Lower.

Where lower?

It shifts around. Mostly left lower quadrant, I'd say.

Now I'm thinking diverticulitis. It's sounding like a classical story. Eating rich, digesting poor.

Any fever?

No.

Chills?

No.

He's a physician. He can do physical talk.

Any palpation tenderness?

Hold on a second.

I imagined him pressing his right hand down into his belly along the soft spot above the cleft where the thigh joins the body.

Don't think so, he said.

How about diarrhea?

Well, I wouldn't call it that. But things sure have changed.

How?

More frequency.

Okay, I thought. There's been a shift in the terrain. Little to go along with diverticulitis. Must have picked up something.

You must have picked up something, I said. Run through the last twenty-four hours for me.

That would be the party last night. Tons of hors d'oeuvres.

Well, that's it.

Food poisoning?

Yeah. Food sitting out on tables long enough, warm enough to be a pretty fine culture medium. Get a little pink medicine, ease up on your diet, and that should do the trick.

I don't know.

Why?

It's pretty bad.

What is?

The pain.

You didn't tell me that.

Yeah. That's the reason I called. I can't even sit at my desk.

The picture morphed — a new photographer with a new camera had just arrived on the scene. What was a simple case of shrimp slush-bucket had become more serious.

You need to be seen, I said.

Should I go in up here? I don't trust the emergency rooms around this place.

Why don't you come . . .

The image of the university hospital emergency room flashed in my mind. A couple hours' wait for a little look at an abdomen that in all probability would be normal by then. It was Sunday night, and I was cooking pasta for my boys. This simple proletarian repast would be ready in about five minutes. They were starving. It was to be a quick dinner, and we'd be loading the dishwasher by the time he hit Marin County.

. . . why don't you come here? I said.

To your house?

You know how to get here?

No, but I'd be grateful if you told me.

I had placed the last dish in the dishwasher by the time he called again, pacing the street with his Mega Light, looking for number 754.

I'll come to the front steps, I said. The lights will click on and show the way.

He sat down. We took a few minutes for him to catch his breath.

It's better, he said. Coming down in the car I thought I wasn't going to make it, but getting out and walking around, it's gotten better.

My couch, sir, my examining table, I said, and with a little slow bow I swept my hand as if before an open door. I gave him the once-over, the usual abdominal exam, kneeling at his side to get just the right angle between us.

No diverticulitis, I said. No cystitis. No masses, tumors. Your appendix . . .

That's long gone.

Even your epigastrium is soft and easy. Must have been the shrimp after all.

Thanks.

I found some pink medicine way at the top of my medicine cabinet, dusted it off, and offered him a couple of tablespoons.

He guzzled it awkwardly at my kitchen sink.

While it was sliding into him, coating him with its simple magic, we sat and talked of other things. We were colleagues in more ways than one. Both of us in our own distinctive manner had separated ourselves or perhaps been separated from the university. I checked in on him.

Things are better now, he said.

Better than what?

Well, you know the story.

There was a story behind the story I hadn't heard yet. Not sure, I said. In any case I liked hearing him talk in that amazing, lilting voice of his.

You know about the growth hormone deal, right?

Tell me.

Well, I'd been working on cloning growth hormone, and we had a fragment cloned that had most of the sequences necessary to produce growth hormone. Then we cloned the full-length sequence. Megagenetics was trying like hell to clone the gene but was unsuccessful.

It's a matter of public record, he said. There was a big lawsuit.

Why?

The Megagenetics laboratory notebooks indicated that they were unsuccessful in December 1978. So on New Year's Eve that year two guys from Megagenetics snuck into the university, broke into the lab, and stole the cloned fragment.

Stole what?

Stole the bacteria containing the cloned fragment. And they

later claimed they'd cloned it themselves to use it to make bacteria produce growth hormone. It's all there in the testimony.

I'd heard about dirty tricks before, but this one caught me off guard.

Yeah. And just think. That was the product that launched the company, *one of the seminal genetic engineering companies in all the world,* and the product that allowed them to go public and make billions.

I am letting the shock waves flow over me.

I've thought about writing a book about this, but it just has not risen to the top of my priority scheme. I'd also have to write in a way that it would not seem like sour grapes.

Why should they think that?

The senior researcher on the growth hormone team at Megagenetics was inducted into the National Academy of Sciences for this discovery, not me. Only twenty years later, when the evidence all came out, did the academy award me with membership.

I thought of all those years he'd been burning up inside, knowing that it was his molecule that had launched a billion-dollar industry for someone else. And that someone else had made all the money and been elevated to national stardom while he got nothing. No wonder he had esophagitis. Burn, burn, burn.

There was a 200-million-dollar settlement.

Must have made you happy.

Not really. I liked the fact that Megagenetics had to fess up to something. Most of the money went to the university, which agreed as part of the terms to name a building after them. They were the ones who sued, and I really didn't know the details until the testimony from discovery all came out. I was pretty astonished. The ironic thing is that when people walk by that multimillion-dollar building on campus, they thank Megagenetics for it. Nobody told them how it got there or what they did.

The money built an edifice with the robber's name on it.

Yup. That's what they did. Built a cathedral.

The one thing that touched me in all this, he continued, was when the National Academy of Sciences was talking to all these people . . . all those scientists . . . they all admitted, every one of them, that I was the one who spearheaded the research that cloned that molecule.

Thank God for that.

He looked off to the side. And his eyes turned soft.

But you know . . . and as that last diphthong-sounding, stretched-out vowel resounded in my head he paused with a wistful look . . . the chancellor never said boo about it.

Never thanked you.

No. Well, I did get a brief message later after someone went to him.

I guess few people know this story, I said.

Apparently.

You *should* write about this.

I'd have to hire a ghost writer.

And I thought to myself scribbler, scratcher, or ghost writer, didn't matter. Any way to just get the poison out of his system.

We just sat there a moment, breathing and digesting.

Some other things have happened since you've seen me in the office, he said.

And with that his tone changed, and he eased off into his other issues, which, stuck between the unemotional phrases, sounded more like attending rounds on the eleventh floor of Moffitt Hospital than any passionate account of his own circumstances. I wondered if he had spent most of his emotional verve burning over injustice.

Little to say, I thought. How time passes and changes or enlarges things. And then I forgot about it. Quiet filled the room, which moments before was not as informed as it was now. I could hear my boys upstairs teasing each other about pajamas. The pink medicine was sliding on its way, soothing some misery here and there. I hoped it would do wonders.

So I should stop by the pharmacy and pick some of this up, he said, holding up the nearly empty and oddly triangular bottle.

Bismuth is a simple molecule, I said. But it does good stuff to the surface of the gut.

He laughed. Simple is sometimes best, he said.

The Pill on the Shelf

I told him to put the Valium in a locket and wear it around his neck.

It's something I might have said, but this time it was my patient talking, my patient the psychiatrist, remembering what he'd said to one of his own patients. We'd been talking about anxiety, *his* anxiety — his mother dying, a rebellious son — how he might need a little something — not to take, you understand, just to have, you know what I'm talking about, just in case.

And I thought of my friend with that paralyzing dread of flying, how just to have the Ativan, not in his bloodstream but in his pocket, was the effect that made it possible to climb aboard the plane, as if having something to turn to, even if he never did, was all he needed.

I like doing pharmacy that way — there's a great and natural appeal to the idea that the only force operating is that of the *threat* of the pill, not the pharmacology of the pill. In that way we can expect all good effect, no side effect. Pretty nice. Fewer chemicals in the body where *our* chemicals, called forth the right way, might give us the halcyon we need.

Once I had a patient with palpitations so bad it scared him half to death. I gave him a prescription for a beta-blocker and told him to put it in the bathroom cabinet and leave it there. Right after that his palpitations went away.

I think that's the kind of idea that ought to pass for national military policy — the best use of an army is to maintain a good arsenal but never to use it. Force and power are best in small amounts, barely enough to set things right again. Then withdraw, allowing the innate rhythms to prevail.

And don't forget that ace in the hole. When the *expectation* we place on the pill, not the pill itself, brings the desired result they call it the placebo effect. So I'm thinking, Let's call that little medicine cabinet phenomenon the Shelf Effect — pretty powerful when the pill works all the way from the next room.

Now don't get worried. I know the limits. When I need penicillin, no imagined substitute will do. And I can't conjure insulin back from a pancreas shot with diabetes. That's just hard science. But as for matters of the spirit . . .

So the psychiatrist guy has his Ativan now. And it was ceremonial. There's just something irreplaceable about sitting down at the desk, writing out the prescription longhand, tearing it from the pad, and handing it to him. He takes it down to the pharmacist, who brings forth this amber bottle with the childproof cap and the twenty-five small white accretions of something wonderful. Ceremony, that's what it is, something about all that, that's just the right amount.

I'm sure he filled it. I'm sure he took it home. My guess is he hasn't taken a single goddamn pill.

Mother Teresa and the Problem of Care

You've got a call from your patient Rodgers who's scheduled for colonoscopy tomorrow.

Memory leapfrogged backward . . .

. . . and hit first upon a different Rodgers, his uncle. The answering service said his first name wrong and led me astray. Right after that I landed on Ricky.

Memory then did another little turn and showed me a picture of him in the office a week ago asking for a prescription for marijuana. He had arrived forty-five minutes late with no apology. After the "how's your family" brand of introductory remarks he said, You remember I have had a little problem with meth . . .

Actually, I didn't.

. . . was in jail four months for breaking parole. That's over and done with, he said. But I've discovered that marijuana keeps me warm, keeps me away from meth, I can stay at home, spend time with my kids, be a husband, everything . . . everything's great, and my wife is happy with me and I'm happy with me . . . so I'm wondering if you could write me a little prescription for medical marijuana, you know, medical in the sense that it keeps me away from methamphetamine.

This was one of those deals whose logic was okay if you just forgot a few roadblocks of reality. Reminded me of the classical description of paranoid delusion — if you believe the pretext, then all the rest follows logically. I had to tell him that, even though he might be right and certainly to use marijuana is far preferable to meth, I didn't think anyone, especially the feds, would buy that idea as a "medical" use of marijuana. And that's not thinking yet about the fact that even though California is culturally accepting of the medical marijuana concept, the feds could put us both in jail.

My parole officer said it would be okay.

Now that was going some. Ricky had a very convincing manner, the kind that, once it got going, assumed nothing would obstruct its progress, no detractions would be large enough to slow it down, no ideas contrary enough to stop it trudging down its very focused path. I had to conclude that that was art. Even I, or, more accurately, part of me, went for it just long enough to seriously contemplate the idea. Then a more rational side bounced up and reminded me of the law, etc. But in the meantime I was, I'd have to say, more than curious about that parole officer stuff. So I told Ricky I'd have to call this guy.

He dialed the number from memory and handed me his cell phone.

The state of California does not recognize the medical use of marijuana, the parole officer said, stiffly. Ricky would be in violation of parole.

Shit! I knew all that already. I couldn't even get medical marijuana for my patients with diagnoses everyone would agree deserved it, but I was so concentrated on the unique nature of the request and the panache with which he had made it that I had soft-pedaled the total illegality of it all.

I told Ricky what he said.

Ricky just said, Okay. Then there was that remarkable deflation, that *pfffttt* of the rush of energy he'd put behind selling the idea escaping out of his presentation. All that strength and determination shut down like a switch suddenly turned off. The most remarkable thing was that he demonstrated no remorse. When he came up against the sharp knife of authority, all the push and surge that would have skillfully carried along the most apathetic or unwilling was suddenly gone. He was used to this. It was part of the game. I was part of the game. Only I didn't know the rules.

Now a new tack: Was there anything I could give him to wash the marijuana out of his system so he wouldn't get busted?

No, I said. And as I did so I got the distinct impression, strangely déjà vu, that I was being used any which way.

Well, while I'm here I want to get checked up fully, he said, all the way.

That's the Rodgers way, I said, remembering how all the other members of his family said the same thing every time they came in.

And that's when we scheduled the colonoscopy, among other things, because he was close to fifty and because I was quite sure I wouldn't get a chance at him for another fifty years.

Memory having now fixed that image of him like hypo solution on a freshly developed photograph now skipped back to Ricky's father, two days earlier.

My son wants to come and see you, he had said. He has Medi-Cal. You don't accept MediCal, but you will see him for me. See him for me. Please, Doctor. You are the best. My son. My son. He *needs* you.

I've taken MediCal patients before. They require *tons* of paperwork. It's basically a pro bono deal because they don't pay and MediCal doesn't either. Somewhere in my office I have a framed check from MediCal in the grand amount of 17 cents, for, as they said in the nice, official-looking letter that accompanied it, *complete and total reimbursement for services rendered.* Government efficiency. The stamp they used to send it was worth more than that. Nowadays I don't even apply for payment — it would be loss chasing loss.

He's my son, Doctor.

I nodded my head. I didn't give him the horror story of

MediCal — that frustrating little song and dance. I just said all right, realizing I was probably letting myself in for something.

Political correctness says not to generalize. Observation teaches otherwise: I knew that beyond considerations of finance, MediCal patients are the ones most likely to cancel appointments, not follow directions, and generally not take care of themselves. Triple trouble. The fact that they are on MediCal sometimes means they have failed in some significant way to make their way in society. Maybe I should be more compassionate. Maybe I shouldn't try to hold them to high standards.

Everybody, even the difficult ones, I was thinking, deserves a chance. Right?

Now he's got me talking to myself.

So this brings me back to the present, where there is a telephone call waiting. I answer the phone.

I didn't prep for the colonoscopy tomorrow, he says.

Why not?

I just didn't pay attention to the instructions.

Why not?

Well, I just looked at the sheet a few minutes ago and it said I have to go to the pharmacy and buy something.

Yes?

Silence.

Well?

I didn't do it.

That sequence of answers would not escape the lips of 99.9 percent of my patients. They would never confess to such a perfectly blatant level of disrespect. Or allow themselves to be trapped inside it even if they were that remiss.

So I'd like to reschedule, he said.

Amazing how some can inconvenience without remorse.

Ah, how do the saints do it? How did Mother Teresa administer to the masses and require so little in return?

Love, they say, not the kind that binds us in pairs or families but love of humanity. Is that it? Not a biological love based on evolutionary principles to produce offspring and protect the young. Something more spiritual, perhaps. Outside the DNA.

Good. But how do I pay overhead, buy supplies, employ assistants to answer phones and arrange schedules . . . create the environment that gets so much done for so many people in one day? A system like this can take only so many hits, and then it goes under.

I was arguing with myself and I knew it.

Ah well, balance, that fine old wine. A little tannic acid, a little fruity bouquet, a little something soporific. Ricky, despite what I may *wish* he would do, will be unable to respond to the "responsible" way of life that we who live "successfully" in society have come to expect of ourselves and of others. He doesn't even feel the embarrassment that keeps the rest of us under control.

So snap out of it, David. You know the score. It's your choice. The decision to admit him to care is *not* predicated upon expectations he cannot meet but upon — what is it? Grace? Something that comes unearned. A gift. A kindness. And that has to be part of the practice of medicine just as it is a part of life.

Like forgiveness in that way, not earned but given.

Tonight I am putting my four-year-old son, Gabriel, to bed. I ask him if he wants me to stay with him or if he wants to go to sleep on his own.

I would be scared, he said.

It's true. And night is when all that agitation comes forth. He wakes up frightened. I have thought it might come from spending his first two weeks as a premature infant in the neonatal ICU, where we could not be with him all the time. His waking up could be a fearful cross-checking to see if we're still around. Since I want to reassure him when the subject comes up, I always ask what he's afraid of.

Ghosts, he says.

Ah, I say. There's no such thing.

Yes, he says. Only in cartoons. Right?

That's right.

Ah, I am so funny.

Yes, but you're a great kid.

Yes I am, he says. And it's good I'm so balanced.

Balance. That's it, that delicate matter. Ricky is missing something. We all probably have something missing. But what's missing from him makes him clash with the general rules. So we have to settle for small celebrations: I will be grateful for his genuine interest in my family, his friendly manner.

Yesterday I had asked my assistant not to reschedule Ricky until I could think this over. I've done that now. Tomorrow I will give the word.

The Doctor's Pill

We were walking back from the Riuniti Bar and Grill in Bronx-ville, writers spent with the passion of writing and all its little exhaustions, several of us who, from the thorough and sometimes ruthless unveiling that writing workshops require, had realized a sudden need to escape for a late-night cocktail. The restaurant had now closed, leaving us to the night air and the unfinished wishes of conversation.

I had been thinking about traumas, how some arrive from a distant galaxy, some close at hand, familiar, seduced by vulnerability. She, no longer sure she was a writer, was even thinking about going home early, on the second day.

We all have our disasters, I said.

I don't believe it, she said. And I could see enormity wrapped around her like a straitjacket.

She had had a hard day. Her piece received criticism, and though it was also praised she heard only the bad things and took them to heart, too deeply to heart, and now I was trying to build her back up.

She didn't want to be built up.

By now she'd already deflected my compliments — I can't hear that now, she had said — and suddenly even truth had no power, for there was no getting by the door of disbelief. And by this she had chosen to inhabit an unreal space, stuck in the unreal, refusing lines of rescue.

Maybe something's wrong with me, she said.

What are you saying?

Maybe there's something wrong with me. Maybe I need tougher skin.

I took a deep breath. Maybe, I said. But skin isn't everything.

What do you mean?

The cars whizzed through the underpass beneath us, their headlights pushing back the dark. A wake of warm air exhaled upon us.

Our walking, without thinking to do so, had separated us from the others, who made no attempt to close, as if separation had taken place by its own intent, by its own purpose, and we, the players, had acquiesced or agreed.

How to do this? If she wouldn't accept encouragement, maybe she'd accept the companionability of someone else's flaws of confidence, especially if they eventually led to some kind of equanimity with the external world.

So you think I have tough skin?

Yes.

Look again.

She turned and looked at me. What I see is relaxation, calm. A lot of calm.

That's balance, most probably. Not too much calm, I reckon. You're not the only one who's vulnerable, you know.

I don't suppose.

Message taken. But no change in her weather. Abstraction was not going to do it. Too weak. She'd have to have proof.

I looked away.

When I was at Squaw Valley Workshops I could hardly read my own poems out loud.

Why?

Hugely nervous.

Why?

Not sure. Partly out of fear my work would be trashed — and at times it was — and partly because I always had a little stage fright, which only served to make trashing a lot more likely.

She laughed. And quickly covered her mouth. Oh, she said. Sorry.

Don't be. It *is* funny. You see, one-on-one I was okay. But put me in a group of thirteen poets . . .

I have that same feeling.

Maybe we should blame the poets, what do you think? Those ruthless desperados.

And I raised my eyebrow . . .

. . . then looked away again. I couldn't see many stars in this kind of sky, and I wasn't sure why. Proximity to Manhattan? Mug?

I think that's partly why I went into stage productions, live radio, television . . . stuff like that. Nothing more daunting than the hot mic.

Overachiever!

Hah! Guilty as charged.

She laughed.

But isn't that what we do? Go after our weaknesses with excessive force?

Probably.

I guess it's better than the alternative.

The wind picked up a little, the kind of night wind you would find on the East Coast in summer, warm but humid with the threat of thunderstorm next afternoon.

I think that's probably one of the reasons I'm a writer, I said. What I'm too paralyzed to get across in a small group maybe I can somehow manage by putting it on the page.

Turning weakness to strength.

Trying.

I still think my piece sucked.

My turn to laugh. And apologize. I started to remind her that I had read all the applicants' pieces, that I had chosen hers for the first day because of its strengths . . . but we'd already been that route.

I put my hands in my pockets and found myself walking head cocked to one side, eyes down, feet almost swinging in an arc to their next foothold on the surface of the world, the way my father walked when contemplating a hard philosophical question or maybe just how to build a fence to contain that goddamn cow. It wasn't enough to share problems unless I could show that there was a pathway to a better place.

I'm on medications now, I said.

Conversation stopped. It was a segue unimaginable yet somehow necessary. We both knew what I said was an unprovoked confession. I also knew it was about making some kind of point. I just wasn't quite sure what it was.

But you're the one who doesn't even take sedation with your colonoscopies, she said.

Yeah, that's me. And I'll probably do it again.

I let the particular brand of my kind of insanity linger in the air a bit and then went on.

But this time it's about cholesterol stuff, I said. I pretty much had to do it.

Well, for somebody who practically has a phobia about taking medication that's some deal.

How did you know that?

It's all over your stories, silly.

So now we had advanced beyond the decorous to the really real. So okay. Here we go.

And a turning feeling swirled around me, a rotation off to the right side where the conversation wanted to pull me, to go slipping off some steep incline or maybe it was a large cliff.

May as well not ask, I thought. I was already there. Nothing to do but push ahead, unsure where I was going but excited by whatever it was that forced me on.

So what you don't know is that most of my life I have lived in fear — not rational, mind you, and even though I totally knew it wasn't founded in reality I was still paralyzed at times.

She looked at me with a mixture of "that's inconceivable" and "liar, liar."

I was having second thoughts. Are you sure you want to hear this?

I'm all ears.

Now we're into it, I thought.

In medical school, studying for finals and probably overstressed, I was struck with an attack of tachycardia — rapid heartbeats flopping in my chest like a bass in a bucket.

Sounds scary.

Really scary. And bear in mind that by this time in my training I'd already suffered at least three fatal diseases, let's see, they were lymphoma, rheumatic fever, and, oh yeah, breast cancer!

She laughed.

Yes, exactly, I said. Goddamn medical student's disease. Probably not unlike writer's disease, come to think of it.

What do you mean?

I don't know. And I could feel a quizzical look gripping my face like a claw. Maybe the story will tell us.

So, go on . . .

Okay. Okay. Mr. Fear came in the door.

What do you mean?

The unwanted guest, you know. The baggage of the stranger that is your own baggage, brought back to you.

She looked puzzled.

It's probably confusing because it's confusing to me. Anyway, I started getting afraid to wander too far from a medical center, a hospital. Eventually, I was afraid to travel in a car by myself, to drive 200 miles to visit relatives. The open spaces I had always loved began to look like danger. I was missing something, balance maybe, perspective. The arrhythmia couldn't have been that dangerous. My concept of danger had been exaggerated by fear so strong it trumped any courageous card I tried to play.

Pretty serious.

Somebody needed to slap me in the face and tell me to snap out of it.

I looked to see if I was boring her. Are you getting tired of this?

Not on your life.

She looked back to the others, whom we could see only as shadowy figures in the half-dark of street lights, their conversation mixing in, at this distance, with the sounds of crickets and road noise.

They can take care of themselves, she said. And we turned onto campus.

Why did you get so scared? she asked.

I've always wondered about that. Partly because of some tendency I was born with, probably, or developed from my overprotective mother, but maybe because medical school was such a . . . I paused, looking for the right word . . . well, it was, at times, a bit like an invasion.

Oh my god!

Well, it was a wonderful experience. I wouldn't have wanted to do anything else. But they didn't equip us with ways of balancing all the heavy stuff they were throwing at us. I mean, it wasn't the cadaver or the diseases we read about. I think it was the unconscious assimilation of all that suffering, suffering we were not equipped to handle.

That might be hard to teach.

Probably impossible. My guess is that role models would have helped, the seasoned physician, the one who is *not* consumed with "protective distance," as the interns seem to be, but somehow has incorporated grief into her life without either denying it or letting it drag her down. Someone who has been successful generating a doubleness factor, if you will, an ability to hold both worlds, that of safety and danger, simultaneously without calamity. Anyway, all that tension went unreconciled.

And, therefore, got worse.

Yes, Doctor.

Well . . .

Well exactly. Obvious, isn't it. That was the first big mistake. Not addressing the problem.

There's more?

The second was probably to depend on others to help me out of it when really it was up to me.

The walk was over, but conversation was not. We sat on a bench as if the bench had been placed there for this exact purpose and for this exact time.

Continue, she demanded.

And something about the demand was just right. Curious, how we started out trying to rescue *her,* and here we were, deep into my own interior. I had to laugh. And she was forcing me on. Something about force at just the right time . . .

Others, you say?

I was thinking about southern Spain, thousands of miles from anyone, nighttime in a hotel, the fierce argument that accelerated in the reckless way arguments do when control is lost, how in the middle of it I was hit with an attack of what I feared most in the circumstance I feared most, and how in the calmest way I knew asked — begged was more like it — just for a little time to recover. You can start where you left off, I said. You can keep the anger. Just give me a little space. How she couldn't do it. How she continued to tear into me. And I came to a realization that swept over me like a hot wind off the Moorish plains of Africa: I knew there would be no one to help me. Not now. Not ever. And in that moment the perception I had made of the terror that was swirling around me created a brick wall between us. I could feel it assemble itself brick by brick. And inside that wall, on my side of that wall, I began building myself into a different person. These building projects, there to protect me, led in some way to the end of us.

When the end came my children wouldn't even talk to me. In that time I believed I had become allergic to fish, to wheat, to aspirin, to penicillin and erythromycin. My throat swelled and threatened to close. I lost fifteen pounds living on potato chips and almonds. Anxiety now had a physical face to it, and that face focused upon food and pills. What to say of this.

I must have been silent thinking about this awhile.

Why are you so kind to me? she asked.

Thoughts swirled and sucked into the vortex trying to get into words.

This is what I can tell you, I said . . . that through the little betrayals and the big betrayals I have slowly learned how to make of myself a person who does not have, or at least is not driven by, fear. A person who does not depend wholly upon the opinions or support of others. I had to give up on the notion that someone would be there to rescue me. I had to give up on the notion that I was helpless and just fucking take care of myself. I think it was important to be a doctor in all this. It was important to be a writer. Both immediately force their way into intimacy and into that sacred place where you can no longer live a lie. And there is something critically important about not lying, about facing reality with its negatives *and* its positives, something about that that is important to this.

Are you still afraid?

Not the way I was.

Never?

Well, this cholesterol thing awakened some of that. But it's strange — all those years worrying about dying of a heart attack, and now that I have perhaps a more legitimate concern in that category I am almost complacent about it. Though, I must say, not complacent enough to keep me from making decisions that are best for my health, even if it means taking pills.

Thank goodness.

Yeah. It's quite possible I grew up just in time.

We were silent awhile.

Could be it's still with me some.

What is?

Well, if I'm alone in a distant place trying to go to sleep at night it wakes me up a few times before I can turn it loose.

So you're a companionship person.

Guess I am. Still am. And I suppose I'll never completely get rid of that little fear, but what's left . . . I can manage.

Sorry you had to put up with so much.

Actually, I'm not. The point of all this, if there is one, is that I've been forced to become a more balanced person. Calm, as you say. I measure things more accurately now. And I don't seem to care as much if someone trashes my work.

My arrival at that point surprised me a little more than it did her. And I wondered if by seeing my struggle she could better see her own, the deeper one, the one exposed by that little window of the criticized piece.

Too early to tell, I thought. Hope for magic. Hope I did the right thing. The really good witch doctor puts a drop of his own blood in the potion . . .

We sat on the bench like old people soaking up the night. There was no agitation in the air.

Strange, I said. I get the feeling I might even be a better doctor because of all this.

I can see how that might be true.

Yeah. It helps when confronting the neurotic or the person who's suffering if you've had personal experience that recognizes what they're going through. Useful. Skips the bullshit.

Then should all doctors get sick?

Probably. And regularly.

We laughed.

And then we just sat for a while, content with where the evening had taken us and where it had not taken us, calmed somehow by it all, just breathing the night air filled with its hint of thunderstorm, looking for stars in the nighttime sky.

Afterword | Brilliance

We were comparing leaf blowers, my three-year-old son and I, his Fisher-Price, my Toro. He was asking why his blows bubbles and mine leaves when his mother came down the steps.

It was Sunday. The day before we'd started working on this new idea about his mother going away weekends to do some writing. Work, he called it. Giving it a name somehow meant acceptance. Even so, I didn't know how he'd take to the idea when she was really leaving.

She stops where we sit on the stairs. She is going away, and we face it head on, on the front steps, with our leaf blowers. And there opens a little pause in which we all know what's coming but not how we're going to get there.

Duston takes the lead. I'll blow you some bubbles good-bye, he says. We laugh. Good-bye bubbles? his mother asks. Nooo . . . kisses, he says. And he showers her with a hundred spheres of light.

Crazy the way doctors think they should always come prepared with the definitive opinion. As a father and a doctor I was ready to teach, to cajole, to lead him through what I perceived to be a tough spot in his life. Instead, my son, on his own, through some mysterious act of will, countered his loss with grace. He had not needed me. It was in him all along. And in that expanding moment I felt a separateness beginning, a split diverging in the road ahead of us.

We walked down the steps together, not holding hands, and stopped at the last step above the street. He cranked his leaf blower and made a kiss-cloud for his mother to drive through.

He hadn't needed help from me at all. All he wanted was to

spend a moment with what he was up against, size it up, and then make his leap.

And there we were, standing together on this lip of sidewalk overlooking the world below. Alone, together, in the brilliance of it all.